STUDY GUIDE FOR

FUNDAMENTALS

OF ANATOMY &

PHYSIOLOGY

Fourth Edition

STUDY GUIDE FOR

FUNDAMENTALS OF ANATOMY & PHYSIOLOGY

Fourth Edition

DONALD C. RIZZO, Ph.D.

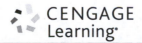
CENGAGE
Learning·

Australia • Brazil • Mexico • Singapore • United Kingdom • United States

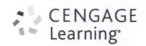

Study Guide for Fundamentals of Anatomy & Physiology, Fourth Edition
Donald C. Rizzo

SVP, GM Skills & Global Product Management: Dawn Gerrain

Product Team Manager: Matthew Seeley

Senior Director, Development: Marah Bellegarde

Senior Product Development Manager: Juliet Steiner

Senior Content Developer: Debra M. Myette-Flis

Product Assistant: Deborah Handy

Vice President, Marketing Services: Jennifer Ann Baker

Marketing Manager: Jonathan Sheehan

Senior Production Director: Wendy Troeger

Production Director: Andrew Crouth

Senior Content Project Manager: Kenneth McGrath

Managing Art Director: Jack Pendleton

For product information and technology assistance, contact us at
Cengage Learning Customer & Sales Support, 1-800-354-9706

For permission to use material from this text or product, submit all requests online at **www.cengage.com/permissions.** Further permissions questions can be e-mailed to **permissionrequest@cengage.com**

Library of Congress Control Number: 2014958906

ISBN: 978-1-285-17416-7

Cengage Learning
20 Channel Center Street
Boston, MA 02210
USA

Cengage Learning is a leading provider of customized learning solutions with office locations around the globe, including Singapore, the United Kingdom, Australia, Mexico, Brazil, and Japan. Locate your local office at: **www.cengage.com/global**

Cengage Learning products are represented in Canada by Nelson Education, Ltd.

To learn more about Cengage Learning, visit **www.cengage.com**

Purchase any of our products at your local college store or at our preferred online store **www.cengagebrain.com**

Notice to the Reader

Publisher does not warrant or guarantee any of the products described herein or perform any independent analysis in connection with any of the product information contained herein. Publisher does not assume, and expressly disclaims, any obligation to obtain and include information other than that provided to it by the manufacturer. The reader is expressly warned to consider and adopt all safety precautions that might be indicated by the activities described herein and to avoid all potential hazards. By following the instructions contained herein, the reader willingly assumes all risks in connection with such instructions. The publisher makes no representations or warranties of any kind, including but not limited to, the warranties of fitness for particular purpose or merchantability, nor are any such representations implied with respect to the material set forth herein, and the publisher takes no responsibility with respect to such material. The publisher shall not be liable for any special, consequential, or exemplary damages resulting, in whole or part, from the readers' use of, or reliance upon, this material.

Printed in the United States of America
Print Number: 01   Print Year: 2015

C O N T E N T S

TO THE LEARNER

You have chosen a career in some aspect of the health care field. By so doing, you have accepted the responsibility for gaining knowledge of the human body's structure and how it functions. This means learning the language associated with anatomy and physiology. Your text and this workbook were written to help you gain a basic knowledge of anatomy and physiology and their terminology. The text supplies the necessary information. This study guide will help you review and reinforce that knowledge.

ORGANIZATION OF THE STUDY GUIDE

Each chapter in the study guide corresponds to the same chapter in the text. The activities in each chapter follow the sequence of information presented in the text. A variety of questions and exercises are included to help reinforce the material you have learned in different ways. Types of activities in each chapter include completion, matching, key terms, labeling exercises, coloring exercises, critical thinking questions, and crossword puzzles. Additionally, each body system chapter includes a case study to encourage you to think about and apply concepts learned in the chapter. Each chapter begins with the statement of chapter objectives. A quiz at the end of each chapter is designed to help you measure your grasp of those objectives.

As you proceed through each chapter of the text, complete the activities provided in this study guide to reinforce the material presented in class.

The following steps are recommended for using this book:

1. Read the chapter objectives.

2. Study the material presented in the text.

3. Listen carefully to the instructor.

4. Take comprehensive notes.

5. Ask questions.

6. Complete and correct the activities in the study guide.

7. Complete and correct the chapter quizzes in the study guide.

8. Review those concepts missed.

This study guide was prepared as a tool to help you learn. The author hopes this tool will help you gain the knowledge of anatomy and physiology necessary for success in your chosen career.

Study Tips and Test-Taking Strategies

Study Aids to Help Enhance Learning

Learning is a process, the process of expanding your knowledge in a proportional manner. Each new piece of knowledge you gain allows you to expand your mind proportionally. How much information have you acquired since learning to read? The learning process ends only with the cessation of life.

Some learners feel overwhelmed at the beginning of a course because of the size of a text and the huge amount of information it contains. Yet, the longest journey begins with the first step. Each word, sentence, paragraph, and chapter helps you learn that which follows. You have taken the first step on your journey to learn about the human body. As you continue that journey, you will become aware of your own anatomy and how your body functions. Use that awareness to build on your knowledge. You carry a "cheat sheet" (your body) everywhere you go. Use it to help you learn.

Reading

It is important to read the text more than once. It is also important that the material be read before it is covered in class. Read the chapter through in its entirety. Reread the chapter section by section. You will note that section headings indicate the nature of the material to be covered and highlight important points or concepts. Note that definitions, explanations, and other emphasized material are usually in bold print. Make notes in the margins, including any questions you might have for your instructor. Sometimes difficult sections can be more easily understood by rewriting the passages in your own words. This helps identify where your problem is in understanding the chapter. After the material has been covered in class, read it again. It is important to note any concepts you do not understand so you may discuss them with the instructor.

The environment in which you read has a great deal of effect on how well you absorb and assimilate the material. A warm room and a comfortable chair are fine for reading a novel or the Sunday comics; however, when reading or studying textual material, it is best to be in a cool room (not uncomfortably cold) sitting up at a desk or table with good lighting. Reading after a hearty meal tends to make one sleepy and negatively affects concentration. Try to limit outside distractions such as television. Pick a time when such distractions are absent or at a minimum. Next, make a short outline using the section headings. Make this outline succinct and use one page for each heading. This is in preparation for note taking that is discussed next.

Listening and Taking Notes

You have read and reread the material for the upcoming class and made appropriate highlights and notations. Now you are ready for the next step in the learning process—listening to the instructor as he or she makes the presentation.

Most of us have little or no formal training in listening skills. There is more to listening than just being quiet and paying attention. During a presentation, it is advisable to take good comprehensive notes. How does one hear, process, write, and comprehend all at once? By reading the material beforehand, making notations, highlighting, and making an outline, the learner has a format with which to work. Good instructors will usually present along the lines of the chapter outline. They will use a lead sentence explaining what is to come next. They will emphasize important points, explain the material, and sum up with a review at the conclusion of the lecture. After each segment of material, they will solicit questions for anyone needing further clarification. Be sure to ask questions if you need help understanding. Remember, the only dumb questions are those not asked. Using an outline will make it easier to listen attentively, process what is heard, and make notes or jot questions as the presentation progresses.

Listening correctly takes effort and concentration. This means leaving personal problems at the classroom door. It means sitting erect and focusing on the instructor, not on fellow students or the view outside the classroom window. Come to class well prepared, having read and reread the material, highlighted, made notations, and outlined; being well rested and having the necessary materials at hand. All this will ensure you are making the best possible effort to absorb and assimilate the material to be learned. After class, you will want to review your notes and compare them with the text to maximize understanding and reinforce learning.

Plan Your Studying

Most people plan their daily activities from rising in the morning to retiring in the evening. When studying, it is also wise to plan. Preparation of the proper materials and avoidance of distractions are a necessity for the formation of good study habits.

Your place of study should be in a room that is not too warm (inducing sleepiness) and not too cool (inducing discomfort). Lighting should be adequate or your eyes will become strained, resulting in distraction.

Do not get too comfortable in an easy chair; instead sit erect at a desk or table. Choose a time when family members are asleep, away, or busy elsewhere. Although some people find music a distraction, others find it helps concentration (if not too loud). Television, on the other hand, is always a distraction. Studying after a heavy meal is a sure way to fall asleep, yet a totally empty stomach will clamor for attention, forcing concentration on food rather than study material. Keep the necessary materials in one place. Having to round up the tools for studying before each session is not conducive to a productive session. One helpful strategy may be to place yourself on an "if . . . then" contingency. For example, if you read Chapter 3, then you can go to dinner or a movie or some other reward that will work for you.

Group Studying

There are pros and cons to group study sessions. Having the ability to exchange ideas, clarify concepts through discussion, and test one another's grasp of the material is often helpful. However, it is advisable to know each group member well enough so that digression and other distractions do not become part of the session. Proper environment, good preparation, and no distractions are a must if the sessions are to be worthwhile.

Workbook Activities and Review

You have read the chapter objectives, chapter outline, and the chapter material. You have read the chapter section by section and made the appropriate notations. You made an outline, listened well, asked questions, took notes, and reviewed the material after class. How can you enhance your grasp of the chapter objectives further? Another step in the learning process is the completion of your study guide activities. They are designed to aid you in retention and reinforcement of the textual material. After you have completed the activities, taken the end-of-chapter test, and corrected all your work, you will have a good idea of how much of the material you have learned. Do not stop there. Do not feel that, once you have mastered a chapter, you can move on without a backward glance. The text is organized to build on previously learned material. However, it is not possible to do this 100% of the time. Go back and review earlier chapters on a regular basis. Use your new-found knowledge every day, if possible. The more you learn and use what you have learned, the more enjoyable the learning process will be.

Using the Internet as a Resource

The Internet provides access to valuable information about the body and anything that relates to health issues. Three sites in particular serve as a gateway to a plethora of information. They are:

National Institutes of Health *http://www.nih.gov*

United States National Library of Medicine *http://www.nlm.nih.gov*

Medline Plus, a service of the National Library of Medicine and the National Institutes of Health *http://www.nlm.nih.gov* (Click on the Medline Plus icon.)

These sites contain links to many other sources of information and should be used whenever you would like to expand your knowledge of a concept or process related to the health field.

Helpful Hints for Taking Tests

There are highly intelligent, extremely well-prepared learners who experience test anxiety to the point of having brain freeze on test day. In reality, we are tested every day. A test is a tool to measure what we have learned; dialing a telephone number from memory is a test, so is cooking a meal, driving a car, tying shoes, and even getting dressed. All of these day-to-day tasks are acquired knowledge and learned behaviors.

Preparation

The first step in test taking is to be well prepared. The previous section presented some ideas for successful studying and helping learners learn. Those steps for studying and learning are the means to being well prepared with the knowledge needed to pass a test successfully.

One way a group can facilitate learning is to have all individuals prepare a practice test on an assigned chapter. Each group member takes all tests, and then answers are checked. Group members find out where they need to focus more attention in their preparation for the real test.

Besides being prepared in the subject matter, there are other ways to prepare for a test. Be well rested; the mind functions much better when not fatigued. Make sure all the necessary materials are at hand before entering the classroom to avoid the frustration of searching for them.

Taking the Test

You are at your desk and the test is in front of you. The first thing to remember is to read each question carefully. By so doing, some answers will suggest themselves during the reading process. The first question is not known, probably because of that test anxiety, but perhaps not. Go on to the next question and the next and so on until you find one question that you are absolutely sure you know. Continue through the test to the end, answering only the questions that you are positive you know. Often the first question you answer will unlock the brain freeze. Then go back and answer those questions you have to think about but know how to answer. Leave those questions you do not know for last. Often an answer to one of those tough ones can be found in another question.

With multiple-choice questions, it is often possible to find the correct answer by eliminating the incorrect responses listed. True and false questions can be tricky. Beware of those that speak in absolutes such as "always" or "never." There are rarely any absolutes.

If you have studied thoroughly, and used your own anatomy to study, for example, using medical terms for your arms, legs, bones, and so on, you can use the "cheat sheet" that you carry around with you.

And, finally, remember this: A test is merely another tool in the learning process. Be prepared, be well rested, and relax.

Chapter Exercises

CHAPTER 1

The Human Body

OBJECTIVES

After studying this chapter, you should be able to:

1. Define the anatomic terms used to refer to the body in terms of directions and geometric planes.
2. Describe the major cavities of the body and the organs they contain.
3. Explain what a cell is.
4. Describe the major functions of the four types of human tissue.
5. List the major systems of the body, the organs they contain, and the functions of those systems.
6. Define the terms *anatomy* and *physiology*.
7. Define *homeostasis*.

ACTIVITIES

A. Completion

Fill in the blank spaces with the correct term.

1. ___ is the structure of the body, and ___ is the function.
2. The four reference systems are ___, ___, ___, and ___ units.
3. The upper structures are considered to be ___, and a lower structure is ___.
4. An alternate term for anterior is ___.
5. An alternate term for dorsal is ___.

NAME: _____   DATE: _____

6. Toward the head is ___.

7. Nearest the origin is ___.

8. The opposite of the nearest point of attachment is ___.

9. The plane parallel to the median is the ___ plane.

10. Dividing the body into superior and inferior parts is the ___ plane.

11. Anterior and posterior portions are divided by the ___ plane.

12. The organs of any cavity are referred to as the ___.

13. The dorsal cavity is divided into the ___ and the ___ cavities.

14. Between the pleural cavities is the ___.

15. The lining of the abdominal wall is the ___ ___.

16. ___ are the smallest units of life.

17. ___ is the liquid portion of a cell.

18. ___ is the study of diseases of the body.

19. The four categories of body tissue are ___, ___, ___, and ___.

20. ___ muscle is found only in the heart.

21. The integumentary system is made up of the ___ and the ___.

22. The balanced maintenance of the internal environment is ___.

23. The body is cooled by the action of ___ glands.

24. A group of organs performing a common function is called a(n) ___.

25. Three kinds of muscle tissue are ___, ___, and ___.

26. Occasionally, ___ is synonymous with inferior.

27. All of the organ ___ together constitute a functioning human being.

28. The ___ system manufactures blood cells in red bone marrow.

B. Matching

Match the term on the right with the definition on the left.

____	29. the belly side	a.	midsagittal
____	30. toward the head	b.	coronal
____	31. toward the tail	c.	ventral
____	32. frontal plane	d.	visceral
____	33. toward the side	e.	diaphragm
____	34. nearest the midline	f.	cranial
____	35. vertical division through the midline	g.	lateral
____	36. divide into superior and inferior	h.	thoracic
____	37. second subdivision of the ventral cavity	i.	caudal
____	38. organ covering	j.	epithelial
____	39. between the pleural cavities	k.	abdominopelvic

_____ 40. separates the abdominopelvic and thoracic cavities   l. medial

_____ 41. cavity surrounded by the rib cage   m. colloidal

_____ 42. solution containing groups of large molecules   n. horizontal

_____ 43. tissue covers surfaces   o. mediastinum

C. Key Terms

Use the text to look up the following terms. Write the definition or explanation.

44. Abdominopelvic cavity:

_____

_____

45. Anatomy:

_____

_____

46. Anterior:

_____

_____

47. Cardiovascular system:

_____

_____

48. Caudal:

_____

_____

49. Cephalad:

_____

_____

50. Connective tissue:

_____

_____

51. Coronal:

_____

_____

52. Cranial:

_____

_____

53. Cranial cavity:

_____

_____

54. Digestive system:

_____

_____

55. Distal:

_____

_____

56. Dorsal:

_____

_____

57. Endocrine system:

_____

_____

58. Epithelial tissue:

_____

_____

59. Frontal:

_____

_____

60. Homeostasis:

_____

_____

61. Horizontal:

_____

_____

62. Inferior:

_____

_____

63. Integumentary system:

_____

_____

64. Lateral:

_____

_____

65. Lymphatic system:

_____

_____

66. Medial:

_____

_____

67. Mediastinum:

_____

_____

68. Midsagittal:

_____

_____

69. Muscle tissue:

_____

_____

70. Muscular system:

_____

_____

71. Nervous system:

_____

_____

72. Nervous tissue:

_____

_____

73. Parietal:

_____

_____

74. Pathology:

_____

_____

75. Pericardial cavity:

_____

_____

76. Physiology:

_____

_____

77. Pleural cavity:

_____

_____

78. Posterior:

_____

_____

79. Protoplasm:

_____

_____

80. Proximal:

_____

_____

81. Reproductive system:

_____

_____

82. Respiratory system:

_____

_____

83. Sagittal:

_____

_____

84. Sebaceous glands:

_____

_____

85. Skeletal system:

_____

_____

86. Spinal cavity:

_____

_____

87. Superior:

_____

_____

88. Thoracic cavity:

_____

_____

89. Transverse:

_____

_____

90. Urinary system:

_____

_____

91. Ventral:

_____

_____

92. Viscera:

_____

_____

93. Visceral:

_____

_____

D. Labeling Exercise

94. Label the planes as indicated in Figure 1-1.

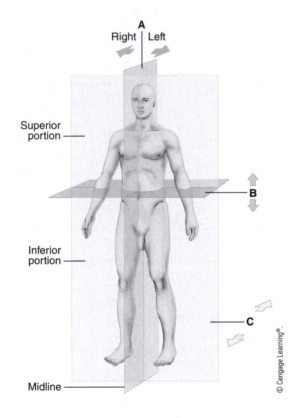

A
Right | Left

Superior portion ——

—— **B**

Inferior portion ——

—— **C**

Midline ——

© Cengage Learning®

Figure 1-1

A. _____

B. _____

C. _____

95. Label the directional terms as indicated in Figure 1-2.

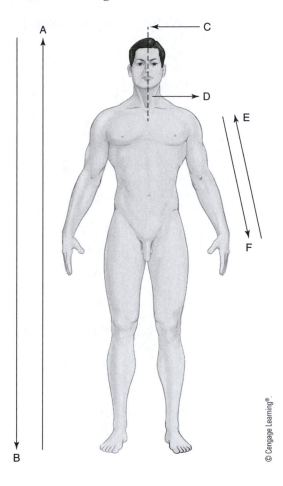

Figure 1-2

A. _____

B. _____

C. _____

D. _____

E. _____

F. _____

E. Coloring Exercise

96. Using Figure 1-3, color the dorsal cavities red, the abdominal cavity green, the pelvic cavity blue, and the thoracic cavity yellow.

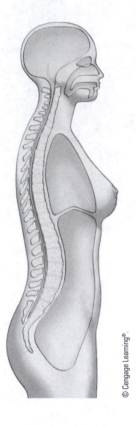

© Cengage Learning®.

Figure 1-3

F. Critical Thinking

Answer the following questions in complete sentences.

97. Why does the tongue have taste buds?

98. Why is it necessary to have reference positions of the body?

99. Why are the mammary glands on the anterior?

100. What do you think a bilateral tubalectomy means?

101. Which system is not needed for survival of the individual?

102. Explain the organization of the body.

103. Explain the "negative feedback loop" as it pertains to homeostasis.

104. Why does our heart pump faster when we run?

105. Which systems excrete waste?

106. Why do we have sebaceous glands?

G. Crossword Puzzle

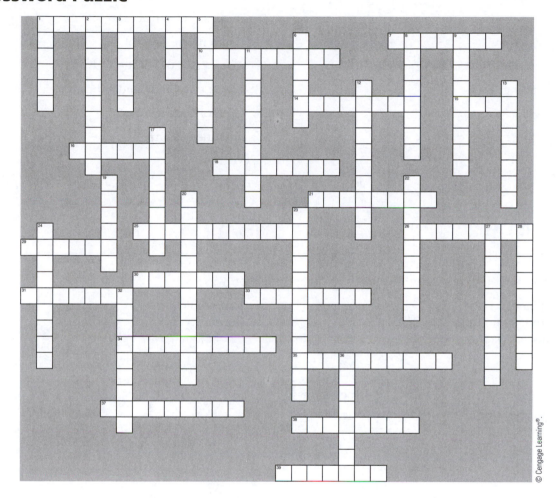

Complete the crossword puzzle using the following clues.

ACROSS

1. A healthy body
7. Internal organs
10. Toward the back
14. Toward the front
15. Basic unit
16. To the tail
18. Cavity wall
21. Cooling process
25. System that brings air to and from the lungs
26. Cavity containing the lungs
29. Produced by the salivary glands
30. Heart muscle
31. Divides the front and back

DOWN

1. William discovered circulation
2. Surface cover
3. Intestinal muscle
4. Senses temperature and pressure
5. Above
6. Farthest
8. Below
9. Ductless gland
11. Horizontal plane
12. Cell liquid
13. Glycogen to glucose
17. Animal starch
19. Back side

33. Goes with superior

34. Function of body parts

35. Body structure

37. Separates the chest and abdomen

38. Right and left parts

39. Blood glucose to the liver

20. Not needed for body survival

22. Studies body structure

23. Temperature control

24. Diseases of the body

27. Tissue that binds and supports

28. Big molecule solution

32. Immune system

36. Nearest

CHAPTER QUIZ

1. The first person to correctly illustrate the human skeleton was

   a. William Harvey
   b. Andreas Vesalius
   c. Claude Bernard
   d. Jonas Salk
   e. Leonardo da Vinci

   Answer:

2. Salivary glands produce saliva, which contains

   a. carbohydrates
   b. HCl
   c. glucose
   d. enzymes
   e. pepsin

   Answer:

3. When referring to terms of direction, the human body is erect and facing

   a. posteriorly
   b. backward
   c. laterally
   d. horizontally
   e. forward

   Answer:

4. The study of diseases is called

   a. pathology
   b. physiology
   c. anatomy
   d. geology
   e. hematology

   Answer:

5. What position is the thoracic cavity in relation to the abdominal cavity?

   a. superior
   b. inferior
   c. lateral
   d. posterior
   e. ventral

   Answer:

6. The term that best describes the direction nearest to the midline of the body is

   a. superior
   b. sagittal
   c. medial

   d. inferior
   e. dorsal

Answer:

7. With relation to the ankle, the knee is

   a. distal
   b. proximal
   c. lateral

   d. inferior
   e. caudal

Answer:

8. With relation to the elbow, the wrist is

   a. distal
   b. proximal
   c. lateral

   d. superior
   e. caudal

Answer:

9. Any plane parallel to the median plane is

   a. medial
   b. sagittal
   c. transverse

   d. dorsal
   e. ventral

Answer:

10. A cut through the long axis of an organ is called what kind of section?

    a. distal
    b. transverse
    c. longitudinal

    d. horizontal
    e. coronal

Answer:

11. A cut at right angles to the long axis is referred to as

    a. distal
    b. transverse
    c. horizontal

    d. longitudinal
    e. coronal

Answer:

12. The body has how many major cavities?

    a. 2
    b. 4
    c. 6

    d. 8
    e. 10

Answer:

13. The dorsal cavity contains organs of which system?

    a. muscular
    b. nervous
    c. endocrine

    d. respiratory
    e. digestive

Answer:

14. The ventral cavity contains organs that are involved in maintaining

    a. feedback
    b. heartbeat
    c. homeostasis

    d. hormones
    e. growth

Answer:

15. The heart in its sac resides in which cavity?

    a. dorsal
    b. coronal
    c. cranial

    d. pericardial
    e. abdominopelvic

Answer:

16. The ovaries and uterus in women are contained in which cavity?

    a. dorsal
    b. thoracic
    c. abdominopelvic

    d. mediastinum
    e. pleural

Answer:

17. The membrane lining the pleural wall is the

    a. parietal pleural
    b. visceral pleural
    c. parietal peritoneum

    d. visceral peritoneum
    e. parietal cranial

Answer:

18. The membrane covering the abdominal organs is the

    a. parietal pleural
    b. visceral pleural
    c. parietal peritoneum

    d. visceral peritoneum
    e. parietal cranial

Answer:

19. The membrane covering the lungs is the

    a. parietal pleural
    b. visceral pleural
    c. parietal peritoneum

    d. visceral peritoneum
    e. parietal cranial

Answer:

20. The basic unit of biologic organization is the cell. Cells grouped together make up

    a. organs
    b. tissues
    c. systems

    d. protoplasm
    e. organelles

Answer:

21. Mitochondria, ribosomes, and lyosomes are considered

    a. cells
    b. protoplasm
    c. organs

    d. tissue
    e. organelles

Answer:

22. The type of tissue with little, if any, intercellular material is

    a. muscle
    b. nervous
    c. bone
    d. connective
    e. epithelial

Answer:

23. The type of tissue having cells that produce elastin and collagen is

    a. muscle
    b. nervous
    c. hair
    d. connective
    e. epithelial

Answer:

24. Which type of tissue has cells so long that they are called fibers?

    a. muscle
    b. nervous
    c. hair
    d. connective
    e. epithelial

Answer:

25. Which system has organs functioning as levers?

    a. integumentary
    b. skeletal
    c. muscular
    d. nervous
    e. endocrine

Answer:

26. Which system is composed of two layers?

    a. integumentary
    b. skeletal
    c. muscular
    d. nervous
    e. endocrine

Answer:

27. Fibrous connective tissue is known as

    a. tendons
    b. cartilage
    c. dermis
    d. fasciae
    e. epidermis

Answer:

28. Interpreting stimuli from the external environment is the function of which system?

    a. integumentary
    b. skeletal
    c. muscular
    d. nervous
    e. endocrine

Answer:

29. Which of the following systems has as one of its functions the elimination of waste?

    a. lymphatic
    b. endocrine
    c. skeletal
    d. respiratory
    e. nervous

Answer:

30. Of the following hormones, which one moves excess sugar into the liver?

   a. glycogen

   b. glucagon

   c. renin

   d. insulin

   e. thyroxin

Answer:

31. Of the following, which is the best example of the negative feedback loop?

   a. eating

   b. swallowing

   c. walking

   d. sweating

   e. watching TV

Answer:

32. Which of the following is NOT a function of the integumentary system?

   a. protection

   b. movement

   c. insulation

   d. water regulation

   e. temperature regulation

Answer:

33. Which of the following is NOT a part of the lymphatic system?

   a. liver

   b. spleen

   c. lymph nodes

   d. tonsils

   e. thymus gland

Answer:

34. Which cavity contains the brain and spinal cord?

   a. ventral

   b. dorsal

   c. pleural

   d. thoracic

   e. abdominopelvic

Answer:

35. Blood vessels dilate to

   a. dissipate body heat

   b. conserve body heat

   c. raise blood glucose

   d. store blood glucose

   e. eliminate indigestible wastes

Answer:

36. Which system includes the sebaceous glands?

   a. nervous

   b. muscular

   c. skeletal

   d. integumentary

   e. reproductive

Answer:

37. What is the thoracic cavity surrounded by?

   a. spine

   b. rib cage

   c. mediastinum

   d. abdominopelvic cavity

   e. parietal peritoneum

The Chemistry of Life

OBJECTIVES

After studying this chapter, you should be able to:

1. Define the structure of an atom and its component subatomic particles.

2. List the major chemical elements found in living systems.

3. Compare the differences between ionic and covalent bonding and how molecules formed by either ionic or covalent bonds react in water.

4. Understand the basic chemical structure of water, carbon dioxide and oxygen gas, ammonia, the mineral salts, carbohydrates, lipids, proteins, the nucleic acids DNA and RNA, and ATP and their role in living systems.

5. Explain the difference between diffusion, osmosis, and active transport and their role in maintaining cellular structure and function.

6. Define *pH* and its significance in the human body.

7. Explain why water is so important to the body.

8. Define the terms *acid*, *base*, and *salt*.

9. Explain how the numbers in the pH scale relate to acidity and alkalinity.

NAME: _____   DATE: _____

ACTIVITIES

A. Completion

Fill in the blank spaces with the correct term.

1. In the digestive process, complex foods are broken down into simpler substances like ___.

2. Sugar is eventually converted into a kind of chemical fuel called ___ ___.

3. All living and nonliving things are made of ___.

4. There are ___ natural elements.

5. ___ are the smallest particles of an element that keep all the characteristics of an element.

6. The nucleus of an atom contains a(n) ___ and a(n) ___.

7. The theory about matter and atoms was proposed by ___ ___.

8. Life on earth is based on the ___ atom.

9. Different kinds of atoms of the same element are called ___.

10. ___ has two electrons in the first level and six in the second.

11. When atoms combine chemically, they form ___.

12. A combination of two or more different elements is called a(n) ___.

13. A(n) ___ bond is formed when one atom gains electrons and another loses one.

14. ___ charged ions are attracted to positively charged ions.

15. In ___ bonds, atoms share electrons.

16. A very weak bond is the ___ bond.

17. Molecules furnishing electrons are called ___.

18. Molecules gaining electrons are called ___.

19. Cells contain approximately ___ to ___ % water.

20. Digestion of food requires ___ to break down larger molecules.

21. ___ ___ contains one carbon atom and two oxygen atoms.

22. ___ comes from the decomposition of proteins.

23. The smallest carbohydrates are the ___ ___.

24. Two five-carbon sugars are ___ and ___.

25. Two six-carbon sugars are ___ and ___.

26. In the body, 95% of fats are ___.

27. Triglycerides are now called ___.

28. Triglycerides consist of ___ and ___ ___.

29. ___ increase the rate of a chemical reaction without being affected by it.

30. The three pyrimidine nitrogen bases are ___, ___, and ___.

31. ATP is made by putting together ADP with a(n) ___ group.

32. The movement through a medium from high concentration to low concentration is called ___.

33. If the solution inside a cell and outside a cell is the same, it is ___.

34. The negative logarithm of the hydrogen ion concentration in a solution is ___.

35. A(n) ___ is a substance that acts as a reservoir for hydrogen ions.

36. Plasma, the liquid portion of blood, is ___ % water.

37. Most buffers consist of pairs of substances, one an acid and the other a(n) ___.

38. Active transport requires energy in the form of ___.

B. Matching

Match the term on the right with the definition on the left.

_____ 39. CO_2 plus H_2O a. RNA

_____ 40. combine with H^+ ions in water   b. ions

_____ 41. move materials against concentration   c. carbonic acid

_____ 42. special kind of diffusion   d. DNA

_____ 43. movement by random collision of molecules e. unsaturated

_____ 44. fuel for cell machinery   f. amino acids

_____ 45. nucleic acid   g. base

_____ 46. structurally related to DNA   h. osmosis

_____ 47. build protein   i. glycogen

_____ 48. fatty acid with one covalent bond   j. solvent

_____ 49. carbon chain with more than one bond   k. atomic number

_____ 50. substance insoluble in water   l. hydrolysis

_____ 51. animal starch   m. diffusion

_____ 52. composed of small ions   n. active transport

_____ 53. medium for other reaction to occur in   o. mineral salts

_____ 54. H_2O helps to digest   p. ATP

_____ 55. ability to do work   q. electron

_____ 56. charged atom   r. lipid

_____ 57. particles that orbit the atom nucleus   s. saturated

_____ 58. number of protons or electrons   t. energy

C. Key Terms

Use the text to look up the following terms. Write the definition or explanation.

59. Acid:

_____

_____

60. Active transport:

_____

_____

61. Adenosine triphosphate (ATP):

_____

_____

62. Amine group:

_____

_____

63. Ammonia:

_____

_____

64. Atomic number:

_____

_____

65. Atoms:

_____

_____

66. Base:

_____

_____

67. Bonds:

_____

_____

68. Brownian movement:

_____

_____

69. Buffers:

_____

_____

70. Carbohydrates:

_____

_____

71. Carbon dioxide:

_____

_____

72. Carboxyl group:

_____

_____

73. Catalysts:

_____

_____

74. Compound:

_____

_____

75. Covalent bond:

_____

_____

76. Deoxyribonucleic acid (DNA):

_____

_____

77. Deoxyribose:

_____

_____

78. Diffusion:

_____

_____

79. Electron acceptors:

_____

_____

80. Electron carriers:

_____

_____

81. Electron donors:

_____

_____

82. Electrons:

_____

_____

83. Element:

_____

_____

84. Energy:

_____

_____

85. Energy levels:

_____

_____

86. Enzymes:

_____

_____

87. Fatty acids:

_____

_____

88. Fructose:

_____

_____

89. Glucose:

_____

_____

90. Glycerol:

_____

_____

91. Glycogen:

_____

_____

92. Hydrogen bond:

_____

_____

93. Hydroxyl group:

_____

_____

94. Hypertonic solution:

_____

_____

95. Hypotonic solution:

_____

_____

96. Ionic bond:

_____

_____

97. Ions:

_____

_____

98. Isotonic solution:

_____

_____

99. Isotopes:

_____

_____

100. Lipids:

_____

_____

101. Mineral salts:

_____

_____

102. Molecular oxygen:

_____

_____

103. Molecule:

_____

_____

104. Neutrons:

_____

_____

105. Nucleic acid:

_____

_____

106. Nucleotides:

_____

_____

107. Orbitals:

_____

_____

108. Osmosis:

_____

_____

109. Peptide bonds:

_____

_____

110. Periodic table:

_____

_____

111. pH:

_____

_____

112. Primary structure:

_____

_____

113. Proteins:

_____

_____

114. Protons:

_____

_____

115. Purines:

_____

_____

116. Pyrimidines:

_____

_____

117. Quaternary structure:

_____

_____

118. Ribonucleic acid (RNA):

_____

_____

119. Ribose:

_____

_____

120. Saturated:

_____

_____

121. Secondary structure:

_____

_____

122. Selectively permeable membrane:

_____

_____

123. Solute:

_____

_____

124. Solvent:

_____

_____

125. Tertiary structure:

_____

_____

126. Transfer RNA:

_____

_____

127. Triacylglycerol:

_____

_____

128. Unsaturated:

_____

_____

129. Water:

_____

_____

D. Labeling Exercise

130. Label the structure as indicated in Figure 2-1.

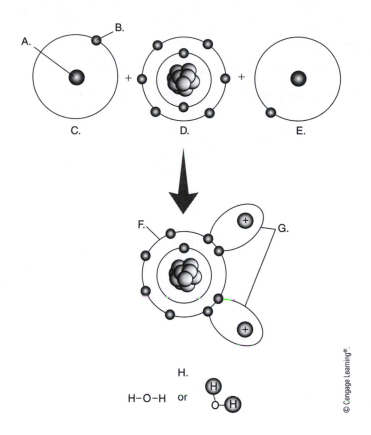

Figure 2-1

A. _____

B. _____

C. _____

D. _____

E. _____

F. _____

G. _____

H. _____

E. Coloring Exercise

There is no coloring exercise in this chapter.

F. Critical Thinking

Answer the following questions in complete sentences.

131. Why do students of anatomy and physiology have to have a basic knowledge of chemistry?

132. Why are atoms never created or destroyed during a chemical reaction?

133. Why are water molecules polar?

134. Why do we not smell ice cream as well as we smell baking bread?

135. Differentiate the four types of protein structure.

136. Why is ATP necessary for cell nutrition?

137. How are chemical bonds formed?

138. Why is the amount of energy necessary to keep some atoms together so high?

139. Why do ionic bonded molecules disassociate in water?

140. Why do we need to exhale CO_2 quickly?

141. Why are animals dependent on plants for survival?

G. Crossword Puzzle

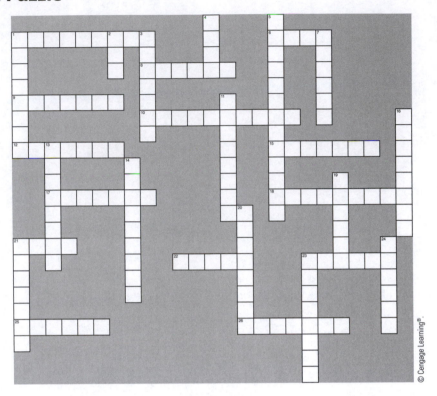

Complete the crossword puzzle using the following clues.

ACROSS

1. They orbit the nucleus
6. Smallest particles of elements
8. Insoluble in water
9. Protein catalysts
10. Basic structure of nucleic acid
12. Table sugar
15. Water through a membrane
17. Adenine and guanine
18. Perfume through air
21. Charged atoms
22. Most abundant substance in cells
23. Found in all living matter
25. Positively charged particle
26. Has no charge

DOWN

1. There are 92 naturals
2. Suffix denoting sugar
3. Medium for reaction to occur
4. Excess hydrogen ion in water
5. Cell respiration waste
7. All living and nonliving things are made of this
11. Bond where atoms share electrons
13. Two or more elements
14. Molecular structure science
16. Normal saline solution
19. Reservoir for hydrogen ions
20. Essential element in amino acids
21. Same element, different atom
23. Needed for nerve transmission
24. The ability to do work

CHAPTER QUIZ

1. The use of water in the process of digestion is called

   a. hydrolysis
   b. osmosis
   c. chemical reaction

   d. photosynthesis
   e. diffusion

   Answer:

2. Primary substances from which all other things are constructed are called

   a. cells
   b. mineral salts
   c. compounds

   d. elements
   e. ATP

   Answer:

3. Atomic theory was a result of a proposal by

   a. Dimitri Mendeleev
   b. William Harvey
   c. Sir Robert Brown

   d. John Dalton
   e. Leonardo da Vinci

   Answer:

4. Atoms of two or more elements form

   a. proteins
   b. amino acids
   c. protons

   d. compounds
   e. electrons

   Answer:

5. Chemistry that studies the nature of the carbon atom is

   a. organic
   b. physical
   c. atomic

   d. inorganic
   e. elemental

   Answer:

6. C12, C13, and C14 are considered

   a. ions
   b. molecules
   c. compounds

   d. isotonic
   e. isotopes

   Answer:

7. A radioactive isotope used to treat disorders of the thyroid gland is

   a. calcium
   b. chlorine
   c. sodium

   d. potassium
   e. iodine

   Answer:

8. A compound can also be a(n)

   a. electron
   b. molecule
   c. element

   d. proton
   e. atom

   Answer:

9. Sodium chloride is a common table

a. sugar
b. protein
c. salt

d. meat
e. water

Answer:

10. Which of the following is NOT a mineral salt?

a. sodium
b. potassium
c. nitrogen

d. calcium
e. chloride

Answer:

11. Weak bonds forming a bridge between water molecules are called

a. ionic bonds
b. hydrogen bonds
c. covalent bonds

d. molecule bonds
e. atomic bonds

Answer:

12. When two oxygen atoms are covalently bonded together, we have

a. water
b. carboxyl
c. molecular oxygen

d. carbon dioxide
e. hydroxyl group

Answer:

13. An important element in ammonia is

a. potassium
b. sulfur
c. phosphate

d. nitrogen
e. ATP

Answer:

14. What percentage of our atmosphere is oxygen?

a. 14%
b. 60%
c. 100%

d. 30%
e. 21%

Answer:

15. Which of the following mineral salts is necessary to produce ATP?

a. sodium
b. potassium
c. calcium

d. chloride
e. phosphate

Answer:

16. Which of the following is a disaccharide?

a. glycogen
b. glucose
c. ribose

d. sucrose
e. fructose

Answer:

17. Which of the following is NOT a lipid?

    a. glucose
    b. fats
    c. phospholipid
    d. steroids
    e. prostaglandin

Answer:

18. Bonds formed between different amino acids to make protein are

    a. ionic
    b. hydrogen
    c. peptide
    d. carboxyl
    e. lipid

Answer:

19. Chemical reactions would not occur in cells without

    a. enzymes
    b. lipids
    c. amines
    d. sodium
    e. acid

Answer:

20. RNA molecules are a single chain of

    a. mineral
    b. nucleotides
    c. glycerol
    d. amines
    e. purines

Answer:

21. Which of the following is NOT a part of a DNA molecule?

    a. adenine
    b. cytosine
    c. uracil
    d. thymine
    e. guanine

Answer:

22. The energy of the ATP molecule is stored in which phosphate group?

    a. first/second
    b. second/third
    c. third/fourth
    d. fourth/fifth
    e. fifth/sixth

Answer:

23. Which of the following is NOT a method of passing materials through a cell membrane?

    a. diffusion
    b. hydrolysis
    c. active transport
    d. osmosis
    e. none of the above

Answer:

24. Random collision of diffusing molecules is known as

    a. haversian canal
    b. down flow
    c. Brownian movement
    d. Hook's movement
    e. Monk's movement

Answer:

25. A normal saline solution is

    a. hypertonic
    b. isotonic
    c. sweet

    d. ionic
    e. hypotonic

Answer:

26. Pure water has a pH of

    a. 8
    b. 10
    c. 0.08

    d. 7
    e. 6

Answer:

27. A substance that combines with H^+ ions in water is a(n)

    a. buffer
    b. base
    c. acid

    d. alkaloid
    e. hydroxyl

Answer:

28. A substance that donates H^+ ions to a solution is a(n)

    a. buffer
    b. base
    c. acid

    d. alkaloid
    e. hydroxyl

Answer:

29. Which is more acidic?

    a. blood
    b. urine
    c. gastric juice

    d. tomato juice
    e. milk

Answer:

30. How many amino acids are there?

    a. 10
    b. 20
    c. 30

    d. 40
    e. 50

Answer:

31. pH is defined as the negative logarithm of the concentration of which ions?

    a. hydrogen
    b. carbon
    c. oxygen

    d. nitrogen
    e. sodium

Answer:

32. Glycerol is a simple molecule similar to a sugar except that it has only a _____ carbon chain.

    a. one
    b. two
    c. three

    d. four
    e. five

Answer:

33. Starch, glycogen, and chitin are formed by bonding together a number of which molecules?

    a. cellulose
    b. ATP
    c. amino acid

    d. glucose
    e. ribose

Answer:

CHAPTER 3

Cell Structure

OBJECTIVES

After studying this chapter, you should be able to:

1. Name the major contributors to the cell theory.

2. State the principles of the modern cell theory.

3. Explain the molecular structure of a cell membrane.

4. Describe the structure and function of the following cellular organelles: nucleus, endoplasmic reticulum, Golgi body, mitochondria, lysosomes, ribosomes, and centrioles.

5. Explain the significance and process of protein synthesis.

ACTIVITIES

A. Completion

Fill in the blank spaces with the correct term.

1. Higher cells like those of the body are called ___.

2. Cells without organelles are called ___.

3. The sperm cell has a(n) ___ to propel it.

4. Cells are measured in terms of ___.

5. Living cells were first observed by a man named ___.

NAME: _____   DATE: _____

6. The cell membrane is called the ___.

7. Protoplasm inside the nucleus is called ___.

8. A molecule with unequal distribution of bonding electrons is said to be ___.

9. Compounds that do not readily dissolve in water are ___.

10. Human body cells contain ___ chromosomes.

11. A spherical particle within the nucleoplasm is the ___.

12. The folds of the inner membrane of the mitochondria are called ___.

13. All cells have approximately the same number of ___.

14. In a cell, proteins are assembled from ___.

15. The expulsion of lysosome enzymes into cell cytoplasm is known as ___.

16. Membrane forming a collection of cavities is the ___ ___.

17. Rough ER is a site of ___ ___.

18. The points of collection for compounds to be secreted are the ___ ___.

19. Messenger RNA attaches to ___ during protein synthesis.

20. The molecule that copies codes from the DNA molecule in the nucleus is called ___ RNA.

21. ___ RNA will go into the cytoplasm and collect amino acids.

22. Two centrioles are referred to as a(n) ___.

23. Cellular organelles located on the surface are ___ and ___.

24. Euglena are propelled by a(n) ___.

25. Paramecium is propelled by ___.

26. ___ cause plants to look green.

27. ___ occurs inside chloroplasts.

28. Layers of proteins, enzymes, and chlorophyll make up the ___.

29. Plant cell walls are composed of ___.

30. Carotenoid pigments are ___ and ___.

31. The molecules of proteins and phospholipids in the cell membrane are referred to in their arrangement as a(n) ___ ___ pattern.

32. It is on the ___ of the mitochondria that cellular respiration occurs.

33. ___ is a natural process by which cells in the body die and is controlled by specific genes.

B. Matching

Match the term on the right with the definition on the left.

_____ 34. structure within protoplasm

_____ 35. organelles for photosynthesis

_____ 36. protoplasm inside nucleus

_____ 37. one-thousandth of a millimeter

a. chromatin

b. lysosome

c. organelles

d. Golgi body

_____ 38. attracts water

_____ 39. repels water

_____ 40. protoplasm outside nucleus

_____ 41. dark threads in nucleus

_____ 42. controls all cell functions

_____ 43. contain digestive enzymes

_____ 44. smooth ER

_____ 45. resembles a stack of saucers

_____ 46. foreign proteins

_____ 47. protein makes long hollow cylinders

_____ 48. plants look green

e. antigens

f. chloroplasts

g. chlorophyll

h. micrometer

i. hydrophilic

j. cytoplasm

k. nucleoplasm

l. tubulin

m. hydrophobic

n. agranular

o. DNA

C. Key Terms

Use the text to look up the following terms. Write the definition or explanation.

49. Autolysis:

_____

_____

50. Carotene:

_____

_____

51. Cellulose:

_____

_____

52. Centrioles:

_____

_____

53. Centrosome:

_____

_____

54. Chloroplasts:

_____

_____

55. Chromatin:

_____

_____

56. Chromoplast:

_____

_____

57. Cilia:

_____

_____

58. Cisternae:

_____

_____

59. Cristae:

_____

_____

60. Cytoplasm:

_____

_____

61. Deoxyribonucleic acid:

_____

_____

62. Endoplasmic reticulum:

_____

_____

63. Eukaryotic:

_____

_____

64. Flagella:

_____

_____

65. Fluid mosaic model:

_____

_____

66. Golgi apparatus:

_____

_____

67. Granum:

_____

_____

68. Lamella:

_____

_____

69. Leucoplasts:

_____

_____

70. Lysosomes:

_____

_____

71. Messenger RNA:

_____

_____

72. Micrometers:

_____

_____

73. Microns:

_____

_____

74. Microtubules:

_____

_____

75. Nonpolar:

_____

_____

76. Nuclear membrane:

_____

_____

77. Nucleolus:

_____

_____

78. Nucleoplasm:

_____

_____

79. Nucleus:

_____

_____

80. Organelles:

_____

_____

81. Plasma membrane:

_____

_____

82. Plasmalemma:

_____

_____

83. Polar:

_____

_____

84. Prokaryotic:

_____

_____

85. Protein synthesis:

_____

_____

86. Protoplasm:

_____

_____

87. Ribonucleic acid:

_____

_____

88. Ribosomes:

_____

_____

89. Rough (granular) ER:

_____

_____

90. Smooth (agranular) ER:

_____

_____

91. Thylakoid:

_____

_____

92. Transcription:

_____

_____

93. Transfer RNA:

_____

_____

94. Translation:

_____

_____

95. Tubulin:

_____

_____

96. Vacuoles:

_____

_____

97. Xanthophyll:

_____

_____

D. Labeling Exercise

98. Label the parts of the cell indicated in Figure 3-1.

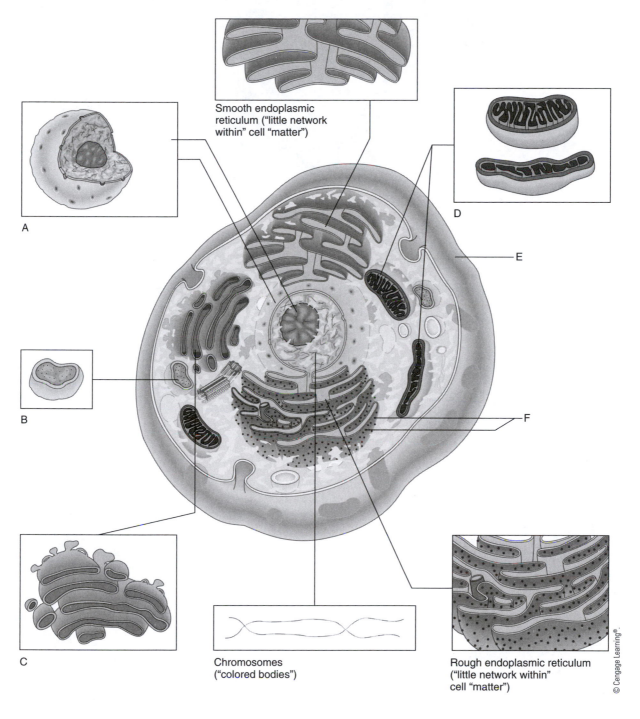

Smooth endoplasmic reticulum ("little network within" cell "matter")

A

B

C

D

E

F

Chromosomes ("colored bodies")

Rough endoplasmic reticulum ("little network within" cell "matter")

© Cengage Learning®

Figure 3-1

A. _____

B. _____

C. _____

D. _____

E. _____

F. _____

99. Label the chromosomal organization as indicated in Figure 3-2.

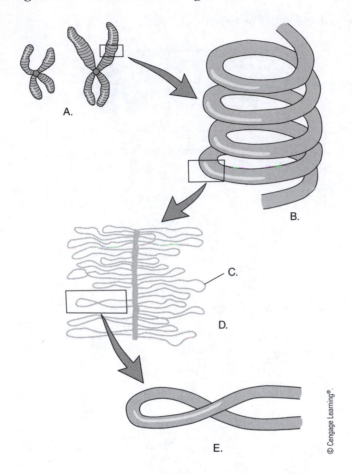

Figure 3-2

A. _____

B. _____

C. _____

D. _____

E. _____

E. Coloring Exercise

100. Using Figure 3-3, color the chloroplasts green, the cell wall brown, the mitochondria blue, and the cyto-plasm gray.

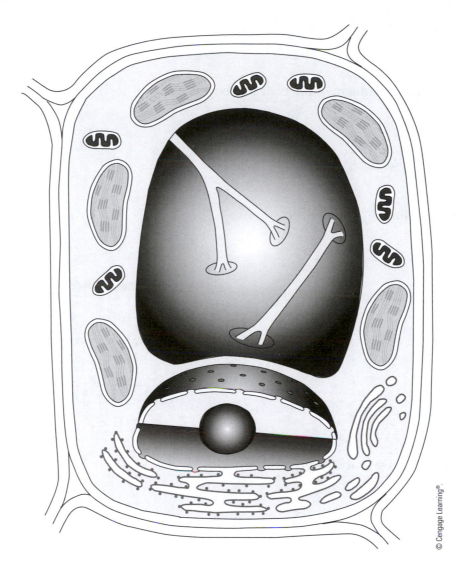

Figure 3-3

F. Critical Thinking

Answer the following questions in complete sentences.

101. Explain the symbiotic relationship between plants and animals.

102. The invention of the microscope was necessary for the development of cell theory. What invention or process was needed before the microscope?

103. Why is water a major constituent of the body and how is it used?

104. Explain the relationship of DNA and RNA.

105. Normal cells contain 46 chromosomes. Which cells contain fewer, how many, and why?

106. Why do muscle cells have mitochondria with cristae?

107. When is agranular ER attached to granular ER?

108. Why do plant cells have a cell wall made of cellulose?

G. Crossword Puzzle

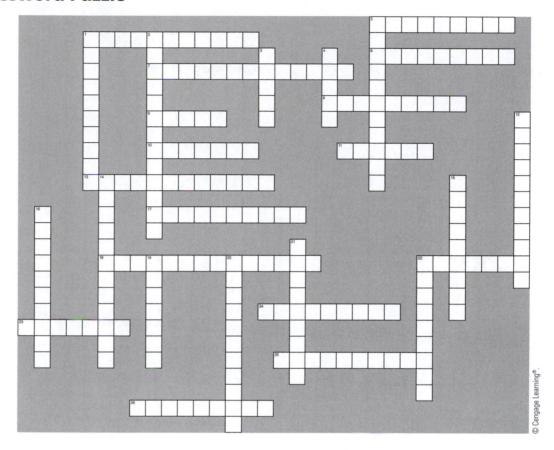

Complete the crossword puzzle using the following clues.

ACROSS

1. Cell membrane
5. Spherical with no membrane
6. Makes plant cell wall
7. Copying DNA code
8. Cell suicide
9. First described cells
10. Control center of cell
11. Stack of thylakoid
13. Plant cell plastid
17. Structures in cell protoplasm
18. Light energy to chemical energy
22. Inner folds of mitochondrion
23. Storage area in cell
24. Contain digestion enzymes
25. No pigment plastid
26. Flat sac-like cisternae

DOWN

1. Like bacteria cells
2. Cell's powerhouse
3. Organelle like hair
4. Unequal bonding electrons
5. Protoplasm in nucleus
12. DNA and protein
14. Attracts water
15. Used in cell division
16. Colloidal cell liquid
19. Long hollow cylinders of protein
20. Matching of DNA codes
21. Responsible for protein synthesis
22. Cell's genetic material

CHAPTER QUIZ

1. Bacteria cells are

   a. organelles
   b. eukaryotic
   c. round

   d. prokaryotic
   e. none of the above

Answer:

2. The most prominent structure in the cell is the

   a. mitochondrion
   b. nucleus
   c. ribosome

   d. lysosome
   e. vacuole

Answer:

3. The first person to observe a living cell was

   a. Hooke
   b. Schwann
   c. Schleidon

   d. Harvey
   e. Leeuwenhoek

Answer:

4. ATP is needed in cells for which process?

   a. diffusion
   b. active transport
   c. osmosis

   d. passage of water molecules
   e. passage of ions

Answer:

5. Which of the following is NOT a function of protein in the cell membrane?

   a. ATP synthesis
   b. pass molecules and ions
   c. receptors for hormones

   d. identity markers
   e. sodium-potassium pump

Answer:

6. Protoplasm is

   a. an organelle
   b. part of the cell membrane
   c. in the nucleus

   d. the liquid portion of cell
   e. a hormone

Answer:

7. Clumps of atoms distributed throughout a medium is a

   a. cytoplasm
   b. molecule
   c. solution

   d. nucleic acid
   e. colloid

Answer:

8. A polar molecule has which of the following?

   a. O positive and H negative
   b. O and H no charge
   c. O neutral and H positive
   d. O negative and H positive
   e. H neutral and O positive

Answer:

9. Compounds of unequal distribution of bonding electrons are said to be

   a. colloid
   b. soluble
   c. nonpolar
   d. clumping
   e. enzymes

Answer:

10. Which of the following would NOT go into a solution?

   a. sodium
   b. potassium
   c. chlorine
   d. phosphorus
   e. none of the above

Answer:

11. Which of the following are NOT colloidally suspended in the cytoplasm?

   a. proteins
   b. carbohydrates
   c. fats
   d. nucleic acid
   e. none of the above

Answer:

12. Which of the following are NOT surrounded by a membrane?

   a. nucleus
   b. nucleolus
   c. animal cell
   d. vacuole
   e. plant cell

Answer:

13. The code to make protein is found on the

   a. RNA
   b. ribosome
   c. mitochondria
   d. DNA
   e. lysosome

Answer:

14. The genetic material of the cell is found in the

   a. chromatin
   b. RNA
   c. ribosomes
   d. nuclear membrane
   e. cisternae

Answer:

15. There are many folds in the

    a. plasma membrane
    b. nuclear membrane
    c. mitochondrion membrane

    d. vacuole membrane
    e. plant membrane

Answer:

16. Cellular respiration occurs on the

    a. RNA
    b. plasma membrane
    c. cristae

    d. cisternae
    e. lysosome

Answer:

17. Mitochondria with many cristae will be found in which cells?

    a. skin
    b. blood
    c. lymph

    d. nerve
    e. muscle

Answer:

18. Maintenance and repair of cellular components is a function of the

    a. lysosome
    b. mitochondria
    c. nucleolus

    d. ribosomes
    e. parallelism

Answer:

19. Sac-like or channel-like cisternae are found in the

    a. endoplasmic reticulum
    b. nucleus
    c. ribosomes

    d. mitochondria
    e. Golgi body

Answer:

20. The site of protein synthesis in the cell is the

    a. Golgi body
    b. nucleus
    c. ribosome

    d. mitochondria
    e. endoplasmic reticulum

Answer:

21. The concentration of compounds to be secreted is a function of the

    a. Golgi body
    b. nucleus
    c. ribosome

    d. mitochondria
    e. endoplasmic reticulum

Answer:

22. The substance that gives plants a green color is

    a. carotene
    b. glucose
    c. chlorophyll

    d. xanthophyll
    e. cellulose

Answer:

23. The substance that gives plants a red-orange color is

    a. carotene
    b. glucose
    c. chlorophyll

    d. xanthophyll
    e. cellulose

Answer:

24. The fiber in our diet from plants is the substance

    a. carotene
    b. glucose
    c. chlorophyll

    d. xanthophyll
    e. cellulose

Answer:

25. Protein synthesis relies on which of the following?

    a. grana
    b. leucoplasts
    c. mRNA

    d. vacuoles
    e. lamella

Answer:

26. During protein synthesis, amino acids are collected. The code for a particular amino acid is made possible by three bases using the element

    a. potassium
    b. nitrogen
    c. chlorine

    d. sulfur
    e. phosphorous

Answer:

27. Centrioles function during

    a. protein synthesis
    b. digestion
    c. photosynthesis

    d. cell division
    e. ATP production

Answer:

28. The number of plastids found in plant cells is

    a. 1
    b. 2
    c. 3

    d. 4
    e. 5

Answer:

29. The process of photosynthesis occurs in the

    a. leucoplast
    b. nucleus
    c. xanthophyll

    d. chloroplast
    e. chromoplast

Answer:

30. The nuclear membrane allows certain materials to leave the nucleus through

    a. pores
    b. tubules
    c. microtubules

    d. vacuoles
    e. cisternae

Answer:

31. The protoplasm outside the nucleus is called

    a. RNA
    b. lysozyme
    c. cytoplasm

    d. nucleoplasm
    e. preplasm

Answer:

32. The nuclear membrane is sometimes referred to as the nuclear

    a. acid
    b. lysosome
    c. cytoplasm

    d. vacuole
    e. envelope

Answer:

33. Chromosomes are made of DNA molecules and

    a. proteins
    b. RNA molecules
    c. lipids

    d. prostaglandins
    e. nuclear membranes

Answer:

Cellular Metabolism and Reproduction: Mitosis and Meiosis

OBJECTIVES

After studying this chapter, you should be able to:

1. Define *metabolism*.
2. Describe the basic steps in glycolysis and indicate the major products and ATP production.
3. Describe the Krebs citric acid cycle and its major products and ATP production.
4. Describe the electron transport system and how ATP is produced.
5. Compare glycolysis with anaerobic production of ATP in muscle cells and fermentation.
6. Explain how other food compounds besides glucose are used as energy sources.
7. Name the discoverers of the anatomy of the DNA molecule.
8. Know the basic structure of the DNA molecule.
9. Name the nitrogen base pairs and how they pair up in the DNA molecule.
10. Define the stages of the cell cycle.
11. Explain the significance of mitosis in the survival of the cell and growth in the human body.
12. Understand the significance of meiosis as a reduction of the genetic material and for the formation of the sex cells.

NAME: _____   DATE: _____

ACTIVITIES

A. Completion

Fill in the blank spaces with the correct term.

1. To maintain structure and function, ___ ___ must occur in cells.

2. The total chemical change occurring inside a cell is called ___.

3. ___ builds and requires energy.

4. ___ breaks down and releases energy.

5. These processes are called ___ ___.

6. The process using CO_2, H_2O, light, and chlorophyll to produce food is called ___.

7. Anaerobic glucose decomposition in yeast is called ___.

8. ___ is the process for adding a phosphate to glucose during glycolysis.

9. ___ is the result of cleaving fructose diphosphate.

10. Glycolytic breakdown of one glucose molecule provides two ___ ___ molecules.

11. The transition from C_3 pyruvic acid to C_2 acetyl-CoA has a first transitional conversion of ___ ___.

12. The Krebs citric acid cycle produces five acids in transition; they are ___, ___, ___, ___, and ___.

13. When yeast breaks down glucose, the resultant products are ___ ___, ___ ___, and ___.

14. During fermentation, the enzyme decarboxylase breaks down ___ ___ and ___.

15. Anaerobic breakdown of glucose in muscle cells produces ___ ___.

16. Fatty acids and glycerol are products of ___ digestion.

17. Digestion breaks down protein into ___ ___.

18. Meiosis occurs only in the ___.

19. A(n) ___ is a sequence of organic nitrogen base pairs that codes for a polypeptide or a protein.

20. Two purines in DNA are ___ and ___.

21. Two pyrimidines in DNA are ___ and ___.

22. The four letters in the alphabet of life are ___, ___, ___, and ___.

23. The cell cycle's three stages are ___, ___, and ___.

24. Strands of DNA duplicate themselves during the ___ ___.

25. The four stages of mitosis are ___, ___, ___, and ___.

26. A(n) ___ cell is an exact duplicate of a parent cell resulting from mitosis.

27. ___ ___ are a group of microtubules between cell poles.

28. Chromosomes first form a ring during ___.

29. The shortest and most dynamic phase is ___.

30. Actual cell division into two daughter cells is accomplished by a(n) ___ ___.

31. During ___, a nuclear membrane forms around each group of daughter chromosomes.

32. The male gamete is the ___, and the female gamete is the ___.

33. Mitosis has one cell division; meiosis has ___.

34. There are ___ daughter cells produced during meiosis and each contains ___ chromosomes.

35. Meiosis resembles mitosis during its second stage; however, there is no duplication of ___.

36. In telophase I, each pole has a cluster of "___" chromosomes.

37. Crossing-over occurs only in ___.

38. The two hydrogen atoms that come off each of the two PGALs go to the ___ ___ system.

39. A congenital abnormality that causes premature aging is ___.

B. Matching

Match the term on the right with the definition on the left.

_____ 40. sex cells

_____ 41. citric acid cycle

_____ 42. defective cells spread

_____ 43. two chromatids, one centromere

_____ 44. cells divide continuously

_____ 45. disruption of DNA code copying

_____ 46. occurs in testes

_____ 47. occurs in ovaries

_____ 48. result in four haploid daughter cells

_____ 49. chromosomes exchange genetic material

_____ 50. full number of chromosomes

_____ 51. forms new cell wall

_____ 52. final phase for cell division preparation

_____ 53. always pairs with thymine

_____ 54. always pairs with cytosine

_____ 55. DNA a winding staircase

_____ 56. two ATP produced

_____ 57. six ATP produced

_____ 58. energy from glucose

_____ 59. nicotinamide adenine dinucleotide

a. crossing-over

b. G_2

c. spermatogenesis

d. diploid

e. gametes

f. telophase II

g. adenine

h. Rosalind Franklin

i. Krebs

j. metaphase II

k. mutation

l. oogenesis

m. NAD

n. cancer

o. ATP

p. $2NADH_2$

q. metastasize

r. cell plate

s. guanine

t. glycolysis

C. Key Terms

Use the text to look up the following terms. Write the definition or explanation.

60. Acetaldehyde:

_____

_____

61. Acetic acid:

_____

_____

62. Acetyl-CoA:

_____

_____

63. Adenine:

_____

_____

64. Aerobic:

_____

_____

65. Alpha-ketoglutaric acid:

_____

_____

66. Anabolism:

_____

_____

67. Anaerobic respiration:

_____

_____

68. Anaphase:

_____

_____

69. Anaphase I:

_____

_____

70. Anaphase II:

_____

_____

71. Aster:

_____

_____

72. Calories:

_____

_____

73. Carcinogens:

_____

_____

74. Carcinomas:

_____

_____

75. Catabolism:

_____

_____

76. Cell cycle:

_____

_____

77. Cell plate:

_____

_____

78. Cellular respiration/metabolism:

_____

_____

79. Centromere:

_____

_____

80. Chiasmata:

_____

_____

81. Chromatid:

_____

_____

82. Chromatin:

_____

_____

83. Citric acid:

_____

_____

84. Cleavage furrow:

_____

_____

85. Clones:

_____

_____

86. Co-enzyme A:

_____

_____

87. Crossing-over:

_____

_____

88. Cytochrome system:

_____

_____

89. Cytokinesis:

_____

_____

90. Cytosine:

_____

_____

91. Diploid:

_____

_____

92. DNA (deoxyribonucleic acid):

_____

_____

93. Down syndrome:

_____

_____

94. Electron transfer/transport system:

_____

_____

95. Ethyl alcohol:

_____

_____

96. Fermentation:

_____

_____

97. Flavin adenine dinucleotide:

_____

_____

98. Gametogenesis:

_____

_____

99. Gene:

_____

_____

100. Glucose:

_____

_____

101. Glycolysis:

_____

_____

102. Guanine:

_____

_____

103. Haploid:

_____

_____

104. Interphase:

_____

_____

105. Kinetochore:

_____

_____

106. Klinefelter's syndrome:

_____

_____

107. Krebs citric acid cycle:

_____

_____

108. Lactic acid:

_____

_____

109. Malic acid:

_____

_____

110. Meiosis:

_____

_____

111. Metabolism:

_____

_____

112. Metaphase:

_____

_____

113. Metaphase I:

_____

_____

114. Metaphase II:

_____

_____

115. Metastases:

_____

_____

116. Metastasize:

_____

_____

117. Mitosis:

_____

_____

118. Mutation:

_____

_____

119. Nicotinamide adenine dinucleotide (NDA):

_____

_____

120. Nucleic acid:

_____

_____

121. Nucleotides:

_____

_____

122. Oogenesis:

_____

_____

123. Oxaloacetic acid:

_____

_____

124. Phosphoglyceraldehyde (PGAL):

_____

_____

125. Phosphoglyceric acid (PGA):

_____

_____

126. Phosphorylation:

_____

_____

127. Polar bodies:

_____

_____

128. Prophase:

_____

_____

129. Prophase I:

130. Prophase II:

131. Purines:

132. Pyrimidines:

133. Pyruvic acid:

134. Quinone:

135. Sarcomas:

136. Spermatogenesis:

137. Spindle fibers:

138. Succinic acid:

139. Synapsis:

_____

_____

140. Tay-Sachs disease:

_____

_____

141. Telophase:

_____

_____

142. Telophase I:

_____

_____

143. Telophase II:

_____

_____

144. Tetrad:

_____

_____

145. Thymine:

_____

_____

146. Tubulin:

_____

_____

147. Tumor:

_____

_____

148. Zygote/fertilized egg:

_____

_____

D. Labeling Exercise

149. Label the cellular respiration steps as indicated in Figure 4-1.

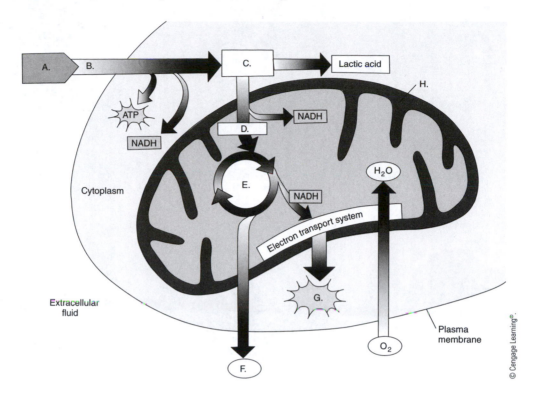

Figure 4-1

A. _____

B. _____

C. _____

D. _____

E. _____

F. _____

G. _____

H. _____

150. Label the mitosis phase as indicated in Figure 4-2.

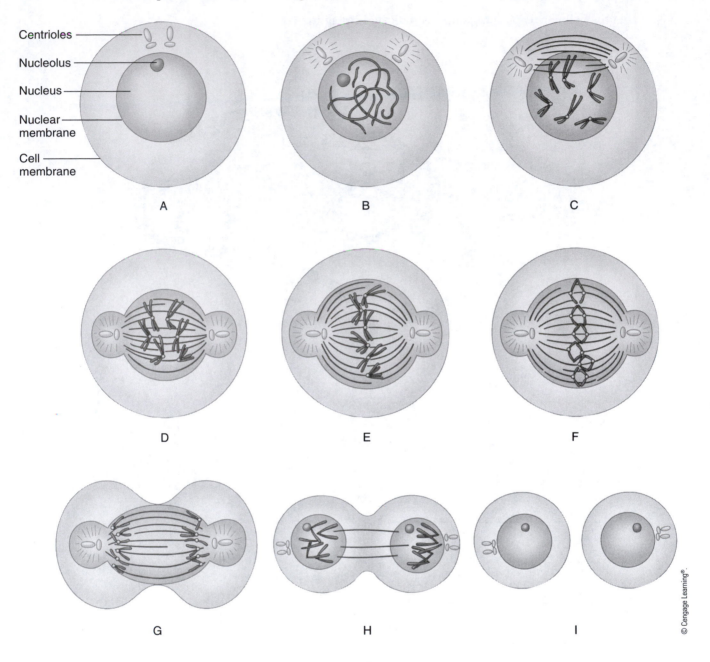

Figure 4-2

A. _____

B. _____

C. _____

D. _____

E. _____

F. _____

G. _____

H. _____

I. _____

E. Coloring Exercise

151. Using Figure 4-3, color the thymine molecule yellow, the adenine blue, the guanine green, and the cytosine orange.

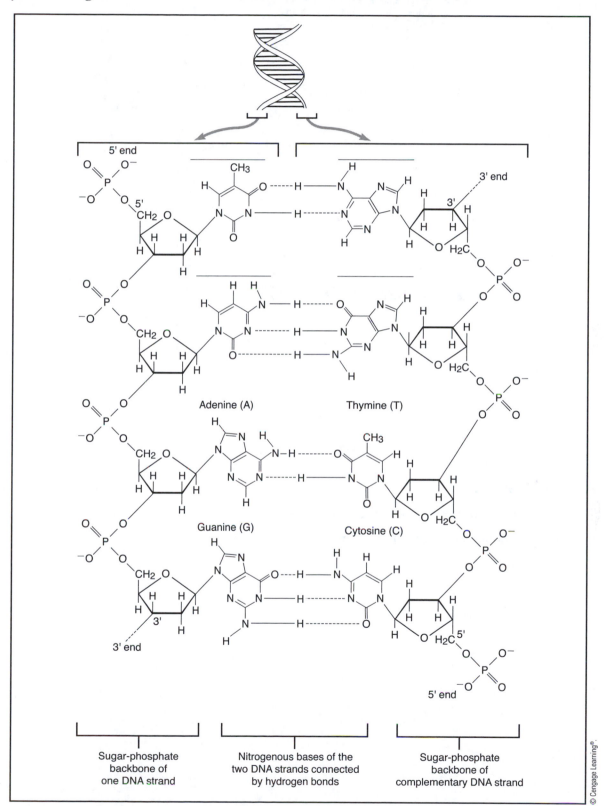

Figure 4-3

152. Using Figure 4-4, color the deoxyribose red. Connect the TA, AT, GC, and CG with their respective colors (those used in Figure 4-3).

S = Deoxyribose, P = Phosphate, C = Cytosine,
G = Guanine, A = Adenine, T = Thymine

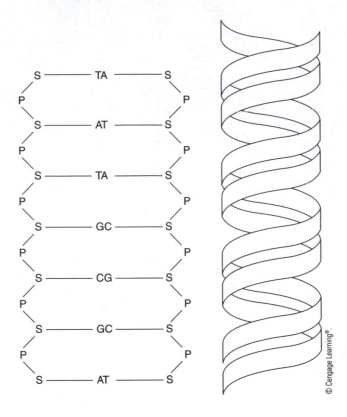

Figure 4-4

F. Critical Thinking

Answer the following questions in complete sentences.

153. Why do we continue to breathe hard after exercise?

154. Why is meiosis necessary?

155. Explain the difference between anabolism and catabolism.

156. Explain the plant/animal energy cycle.

157. Why is the biochemical production of energy more efficient than that of a man-made machine?

158. Why do alanine and lactic acid enter the cellular furnace at the pyruvic acid stage?

159. Why was the revelation of Rosalind Franklin, James Watson, and Francis Crick so important?

160. What is a gene?

161. Why is the genome project so important?

162. Is interphase really a resting phase? Explain.

163. Which of the three cellular reproduction careers interest you the most? Why?

G. Crossword Puzzle

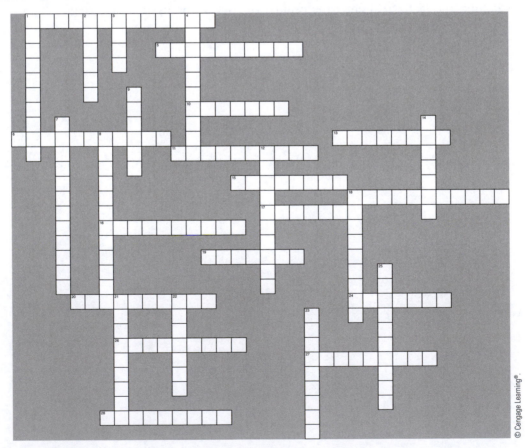

Complete the crossword puzzle using the following clues.

ACROSS

1. Formation of sex cells
5. Cellular respiration
6. Disk of protein
10. 23 chromosomes
11. Pinched in area
13. Friedreich the chemist
15. Disruption of genetic code
16. Phosphate group
17. Bone cancer
18. Organelle duplication
19. Reduction division
20. Cancer causing
24. Normal cell division
26. Formation of female egg
27. Builds molecules
28. Without oxygen

DOWN

1. Cell respiration
2. Visible pair of chromosomes
3. Sequence of organic nitrogen
4. Between phases
7. Yeast cells feed on glucose
8. Exchange genetic material
9. Fertilized egg
12. Tumor moves
14. Needing oxygen
18. From epithelial tissue
21. Dark threads
22. Pairs with cytosine
23. X-shaped structure
25. Break down molecule

CHAPTER QUIZ

1. The complete chemical process of chemical change in a cell is called

   a. anabolism
   b. metabolism
   c. catabolism
   d. glycolysis
   e. digestion

Answer:

2. Breaking down molecules with a release of energy is

   a. anabolism
   b. metabolism
   c. catabolism
   d. glycolysis
   e. digestion

Answer:

3. Using energy to construct molecular material is

   a. anabolism
   b. metabolism
   c. catabolism
   d. glycolysis
   e. digestion

Answer:

4. The ultimate source of food is the result of a process called

   a. metabolism
   b. glycolysis
   c. photosynthesis
   d. aerobics
   e. mitosis

Answer:

5. Which of the following is NOT used in photosynthesis?

   a. H_2O
   b. $6CO_2$
   c. light
   d. chlorophyll
   e. O_2

Answer:

6. The first step in the process of breaking down a glucose molecule is

   a. digestion
   b. aerobic
   c. anabolism
   d. glycolysis
   e. photosynthesis

Answer:

7. During the latter part of prolonged exercise, human muscles start to break down glucose by the process of

   a. anaerobic respiration
   b. aerobic respiration
   c. respiration
   d. anabolism
   e. electron transport

Answer:

8. During glycolysis, glucose is broken down to

   a. lactic acid
   b. malic acid
   c. pyruvic acid
   d. citric acid
   e. folic acid

Answer:

9. Phosphoglyceric acid is formed in which step of glycolysis?

   a. first
   b. second
   c. third
   d. fourth
   e. fifth

Answer:

10. When the phosphoglyceric acids are broken down, how many ATP molecules are formed?

   a. 2
   b. 4
   c. 6
   d. 8
   e. 10

Answer:

11. Aerobic glycolysis produces how many molecules of ATP?

   a. 2
   b. 4
   c. 6
   d. 8
   e. 10

Answer:

12. During the first part of the Krebs citric acid cycle, pyruvic acid is converted to

    a. acetic acid
    b. lactic acid
    c. oxaloacetic acid

    d. malic acid
    e. succinic acid

Answer:

13. The Krebs citric acid cycle takes place in the

    a. lysosome
    b. vacuoles
    c. nucleus

    d. mitochondria
    e. ribosomes

Answer:

14. Alpha-ketoglutaric acid is broken down into

    a. malic acid
    b. pyruvic acid
    c. acetic acid

    d. succinic acid
    e. folic acid

Answer:

15. The electrons of which element are the primary substance carried by the electron transport system?

    a. hydrogen
    b. oxygen
    c. phosphorus

    d. sulfur
    e. potassium

Answer:

16. The final product of fermentation is

    a. malic acid
    b. alcohol
    c. yeast

    d. sugar
    e. bread

Answer:

17. During anaerobic production of ATP in muscle, which acid is formed?

    a. pyruvic
    b. folic
    c. malic

    d. oxaloacetic
    e. lactic

Answer:

18. Which of the following is NOT a carbohydrate?

    a. glucose
    b. starch
    c. glycogen

    d. monosaccharides
    e. glycerol

Answer:

19. The actual separation of the cell into two daughter cells is called

    a. cytokinesis
    b. mitosis
    c. meiosis

    d. phosphorylation
    e. catabolism

Answer:

20. The two purines are composed of

    a. folic acid and oxygen
    b. thymine and cytosine
    c. adenine and guanine

    d. cytosine and adenine
    e. adenine and thymine

Answer:

21. The two pyrimidines are composed of

    a. folic acid and oxygen
    b. thymine and cytosine
    c. adenine and guanine

    d. cytosine and adenine
    e. adenine and thymine

Answer:

22. Certain cells divide only if damaged; they are

    a. skin cells
    b. hair cells
    c. liver cells

    d. blood cells
    e. muscle cells

Answer:

23. The longest phase of the cell cycle is

    a. prophase
    b. telophase
    c. cytokinesis

    d. interphase
    e. mitosis

Answer:

24. Which of the following is NOT a stage of mitosis?

    a. interphase
    b. prophase
    c. metaphase

    d. anaphase
    e. telophase

Answer:

25. Which of the following is NOT part of prophase?

    a. aster
    b. kinetochore
    c. centromere

    d. spindle fiber
    e. none of the above

Answer:

26. All of the following are a part of metaphase EXCEPT

    a. aster
    b. kinetochore
    c. centromere

    d. spindle fiber
    e. none of the above

Answer:

27. Which of the following is the shortest phase of mitosis?

    a. interphase
    b. prophase
    c. metaphase

    d. anaphase
    e. telophase

Answer:

28. The final stage of mitosis is

    a. interphase
    b. telophase
    c. prophase

    d. anaphase
    e. metaphase

Answer:

29. A cell with 23 chromosomes is

    a. diploid
    b. muscle
    c. zygote

    d. haploid
    e. gonad

Answer:

30. Which of the following cancers is considered hereditary?

    a. colon
    b. lung
    c. skin

    d. breast
    e. none of the above

Answer:

31. The second stage of mitosis is

    a. metaphase
    b. anaphase
    c. cytokinesis

    d. telophase
    e. prophase

Answer:

32. In the citric acid cycle, citric acid is formed from acetyl-CoA reacting with which of the following?

    a. oxaloacetic acid
    b. acetic acid
    c. carbonic acid

    d. PGAL
    e. glucose

Answer:

33. Which of the following professionals establish daily balanced dietary intakes for individuals?

    a. cell biologists
    b. gerontologists
    c. dieticians

    d. genetic engineers
    e. consultants in planned parenthood

Answer:

Tissues

ACTIVITIES

A. Completion

Fill in the blank spaces with the correct term.

1. One who specializes in analyzing tissue samples looking for clues that help solve crimes is a(n) ___ ___.

2. Groups of cells with similar function form ___.

3. The four types of tissue in the human body are ___, ___, ___, and ___.

4. The four functions of epithelial tissue are ___, ___, ___, and ___.

NAME: _____   DATE: _____

5. Tall and rectangular cells are called ___.

6. A simple arrangement of epithelial cells can be found in the ___, ___, and ___.

7. The epithelial cell arrangement found lining the throat is called ___.

8. Mucous membranes are usually ___.

9. Glandular tissue forms ___ and ___ glands.

10. The tissue lining the circulatory system is ___.

11. The mesothelium is also called ___ tissue.

12. The type of tissue providing for movement and support is ___.

13. This type of tissue has intercellular material called a(n) ___.

14. Connective tissue has the subgroups called ___, ___, and ___.

15. The most widely distributed connective tissue is ___.

16. Areolar tissue has three main types of cells, ___, ___, and ___ cells.

17. ___ tissue is fat.

18. Dense connective tissues bearing a regular arrangement of fibers are ___.

19. The connective tissue attaching bones to bones is called ___.

20. The tissue covering a muscle is ___.

21. Cells of cartilage are called ___.

22. Cartilage that has a matrix with no fibers is called ___.

23. Elastin fibers embedded in the matrix of this connective tissue give it the name ___ cartilage.

24. The dense connective tissue making up the teeth is named ___.

25. ___ is liquid tissue.

26. Mucus-secreting tissues are made up of ___ cells.

27. Marrow and lymphoid organs are referred to as ___ tissue.

28. Phagocytes are found in ____ tissue.

29. Three types of muscle tissue are ___, ___, and ___.

30. A neuron consists of a(n) ___, a(n) ___ ___, and a(n) ___.

31. If exposed to repeated irritation, other epithelial cells can become ___ in appearance.

32. The two types of exocrine glands are ___ and ___.

33. The intervertebral disks that surround the spinal cord are made of ___.

B. Matching

Match the term on the right with the definition on the left.

____ 34. study of tissue   a. heparin

____ 35. cells flat and irregular   b. Kupffer's

____ 36. small cubes   c. cardiac

____ 37. secrete mucus   d. histology

____ 38. lines thoracic cavity   e. muscle tissue

_____ 39. lines abdominal cavity

_____ 40. motile phagocytes

_____ 41. anticoagulant

_____ 42. wide flat tendon

_____ 43. cartilage cavities

_____ 44. cells lining liver

_____ 45. phagocytic cell in nervous system

_____ 46. ability to shorten and thicken

_____ 47. pushes food along digestive tract

_____ 48. striated muscle

_____ 49. cells shorter than smooth

_____ 50. ductless glands

_____ 51. make fibers for repair

_____ 52. intervertebral disks

_____ 53. conducting cells

f. lacunae

g. squamous

h. fibroblasts

i. cuboidal

j. pleura

k. endocrine

l. neurons

m. peritoneum

n. goblet cells

o. fibrocartilage

p. aponeurosis

q. neuroglia

r. skeletal

s. macrophages

t. peristalsis

C. Key Terms

Use the text to look up the following terms. Write the definition or explanation.

54. Adipose:

_____

_____

55. Aponeuroses:

_____

_____

56. Areolar:

_____

_____

57. Axon:

_____

_____

58. Axon endings:

_____

_____

59. Basement membrane:

_____

_____

60. Blood:

_____

_____

61. Bone:

_____

_____

62. Cancellous bone:

_____

_____

63. Cardiac muscle:

_____

_____

64. Cell body:

_____

_____

65. Chondrocyte:

_____

_____

66. Collagen:

_____

_____

67. Columnar epithelium:

_____

_____

68. Compact bone:

_____

_____

69. Compound exocrine glands:

_____

_____

70. Connective tissue:

_____

_____

71. Cuboidal epithelium:

_____

_____

72. Dendrite:

_____

_____

73. Dentin:

_____

_____

74. Elastin:

_____

_____

75. Elastic cartilage:

_____

_____

76. Endocardium:

_____

_____

77. Endocrine glands:

_____

_____

78. Endothelium:

_____

_____

79. Epithelial tissue:

_____

_____

80. Erythrocytes:

_____

_____

81. Exocrine glands:

_____

_____

82. Fascia:

_____

_____

83. Fibroblasts:

_____

_____

84. Fibrocartilage:

_____

_____

85. Glandular epithelium:

_____

_____

86. Goblet cells:

_____

_____

87. Hematopoietic tissue:

_____

_____

88. Heparin:

_____

_____

89. Histamine:

_____

_____

90. Histiocytes:

_____

_____

91. Histology:

_____

_____

92. Hyaline cartilage:

_____

_____

93. Intercalated disks:

_____

_____

94. Kupffer's cells:

_____

_____

95. Lacunae:

_____

_____

96. Leukocytes:

_____

_____

97. Ligaments:

_____

_____

98. Lymphoid tissue:

_____

_____

99. Macrophages:

_____

_____

100. Mast cells:

_____

_____

101. Matrix:

_____

_____

102. Mesothelium:

_____

_____

103. Microglia:

_____

_____

104. Mucous membrane/epithelium:

_____

_____

105. Muscle fibers:

_____

_____

106. Muscle tissue:

_____

_____

107. Neuroglia:

_____

_____

108. Neuron:

_____

_____

109. Osteocytes:

_____

_____

110. Parietal:

_____

_____

111. Pericardium:

_____

_____

112. Peristalsis:

_____

_____

113. Peritoneum:

_____

_____

114. Phagocytic:

_____

_____

115. Pleura:

_____

_____

116. Pseudostratified epithelial:

_____

_____

117. Reticular:

_____

_____

118. Reticuloendothelial system:

_____

_____

119. Serous tissue:

_____

_____

120. Simple epithelial:

_____

_____

121. Simple exocrine glands:

_____

_____

122. Smooth muscle:

_____

_____

123. Squamous epithelium:

_____

_____

124. Stratified epithelial:

_____

_____

125. Striated muscle:

_____

_____

126. Synovial membrane:

_____

_____

127. Tendons:

_____

_____

128. Tissue:

_____

_____

129. Transitional epithelial:

_____

_____

130. Visceral:

_____

_____

D. Labeling Exercise

131. Label Figure 5-1 as indicated.

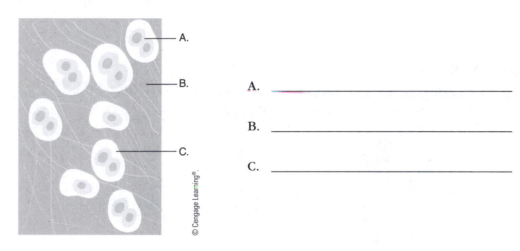

A. _____

B. _____

C. _____

Figure 5-1

132. Label Figure 5-2 as indicated.

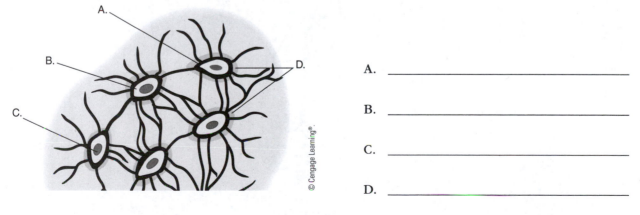

A. _____

B. _____

C. _____

D. _____

Figure 5-2

133. Label Figure 5-3 as indicated.

A. _____

B. _____

C. _____

D. _____

Figure 5-3

E. Coloring Exercise

134. Using Figure 5-4, color the erythrocytes red, thrombocytes green, lymphocyte blue, neutrophil yellow, monocyte brown, basophil orange, and eosinophil pink.

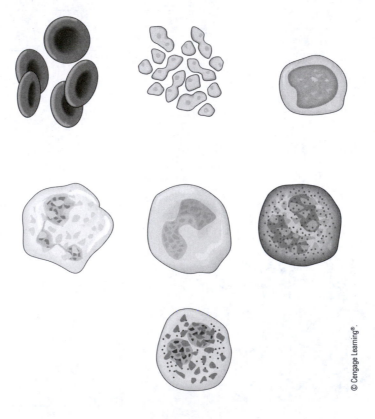

Figure 5-4

F. Critical Thinking

Answer the following questions in complete sentences.

135. Why is the basement membrane important?

136. Explain the versatility of epithelial tissue.

137. Why is transitional epithelial tissue important?

138. Explain the functions of the mucous membrane.

139. Give an example of a simple and a complex exocrine gland, and state the function of your example.

140. Why would heparin be important to the body?

141. Would an obese person be more or less sensitive to temperature change?

142. How are macrophages a help to the protection of the body?

143. In general, how do muscles work?

144. How will nervous tissue help you pass this course?

145. Why do injuries in older adults heal more slowly?

G. Crossword Puzzle

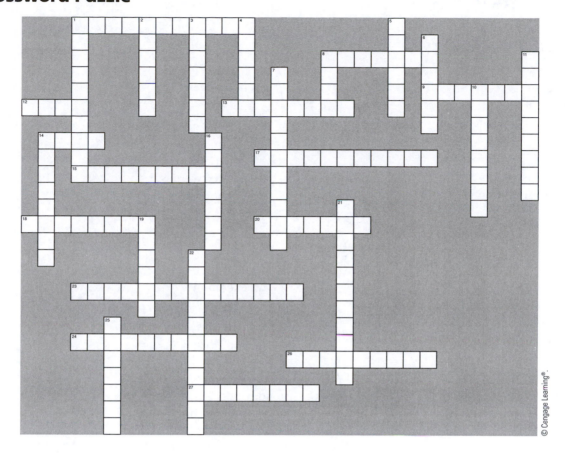

Complete the crossword puzzle using the following clues.

ACROSS

1. Lines circulatory system
8. Fat cells
9. Attach muscle to bone
12. Firm, specialized connective tissue
13. Sweat glands
14. Epithelial tissue protecting underlying tissue
15. Phagocytes in the CNS
17. Wide flat tendon
18. Fiber in matrix
20. Made by mast cells
23. Collagenous fiber in matrix
24. Cells that eat debris
26. Study of tissue
27. Skeletal muscle

DOWN

1. Simple arrangement is one cell thick
2. Groups of cells
3. Cavities in a firm matrix
4. Intercellular material
5. Involuntary muscle tissue
6. Teeth material
7. Motile phagocytes
8. Transmits a nerve impulse
10. Receives and conducts stimuli
11. Produced in response to allergies
12. Flat, irregularly shaped cells
16. Matrix with no visible fibers
19. Nerve cell
21. Forms fibrils
22. Pushes material by muscle contraction
25. Muscle of heart

CHAPTER QUIZ

1. Histology is the study of

   a. cells
   b. organs
   c. tissues

   d. disease
   e. organelles

   Answer:

2. A histiocyte is a cell in

   a. nervous tissue
   b. epithelial tissue
   c. muscle tissue

   d. connective tissue
   e. blood tissue

   Answer:

3. All of the following are functions of epithelial tissue EXCEPT

   a. movement
   b. secretion
   c. protection

   d. excretion
   e. absorption

   Answer:

4. Which tissue has little intercellular material?

   a. loose connective
   b. dense connective
   c. epithelial

   d. specialized connective
   e. none of the above

   Answer:

5. Kupffer's cells are found in the

   a. heart
   b. bladder
   c. liver

   d. teeth
   e. brain

   Answer:

6. Which are cuboidal cells?

   a. pancreas
   b. liver
   c. brain

   d. teeth
   e. ovaries

   Answer:

7. The membrane lining the lungs is the

   a. parietal peritoneum
   b. visceral peritoneum
   c. parietal pleural

   d. visceral pleural
   e. basement

   Answer:

8. The lining of the blood vessels is made up of

   a. cuboidal cells
   b. squamous cells
   c. columnar cells

   d. muscle cells
   e. nervous cells

   Answer:

9. Alveoli of the lungs have which kind of cell arrangement?

   a. pseudostratified
   b. stratified
   c. transitional

   d. simple
   e. common

Answer:

10. If it is relaxed tissue and the cell layer looks like the teeth of a saw, it is

    a. transitional
    b. stratified
    c. common

    d. pseudostratified
    e. simple

Answer:

11. Glandular epithelial forms the following types of glands EXCEPT

    a. salivary
    b. sweat
    c. gallbladder

    d. mammary
    e. sebaceous

Answer:

12. Which glands are unicellular?

    a. tear
    b. endocrine
    c. goblet

    d. simple exocrine
    e. compound exocrine

Answer:

13. The vessels made up of endothelium in a simple cell arrangement are

    a. capillaries
    b. arterioles
    c. arteries

    d. vessels
    e. veins

Answer:

14. Serous tissue does NOT

    a. protect
    b. excrete
    c. reduce friction

    d. secrete
    e. none of the above

Answer:

15. Types of connective tissue are cells of the following EXCEPT

    a. loose
    b. areolar
    c. dense

    d. endocardial
    e. specialized

Answer:

16. A type of loose connective tissue is

    a. tendon
    b. blood
    c. areolar

    d. lymphoid
    e. fibrocartilage

Answer:

17. The tissue that makes up the subcutaneous layer is

    a. adipose
    b. areolar
    c. hyaline

    d. reticular
    e. specialized

Answer:

18. Chondrocytes are found in

    a. bone
    b. blood
    c. muscle

    d. cartilage
    e. epithelial tissue

Answer:

19. The cartilage with tough collagenous fibers is

    a. hyaline
    b. tendons
    c. aponeurosis

    d. fibrocartilage
    e. elastic

Answer:

20. Which of the following is NOT an example of specialized connective tissue?

    a. dentin
    b. fat
    c. bone

    d. blood
    e. lymphoid

Answer:

21. Kupffer's cells, macrophages, and neuroglia make up the

    a. reticuloendothelial system
    b. mast system
    c. lymph system

    d. sensory system
    e. nervous system

Answer:

22. Synovial membranes line joints and

    a. vessels
    b. bursae
    c. tendons

    d. ligaments
    e. aponeurosis

Answer:

23. Synovial membranes function in

    a. temperature control
    b. protection from disease
    c. absorption

    d. excretion
    e. friction reduction

Answer:

24. Which tissue functions as an insulator?

    a. elastic
    b. dense
    c. hyaline

    d. adipose
    e. loose

Answer:

25. Muscles have the ability to shorten and thicken due to

    a. amine and cytosine
    b. actin and cytosine
    c. hyaline and myosin
    d. actin and myosin
    e. none of the above

Answer:

26. Of the three muscle types—smooth, striated, and cardiac—only striated is

    a. voluntary
    b. involuntary
    c. peristaltic
    d. spindle-shaped
    e. uninucleated

Answer:

27. The muscle attached to bones is

    a. smooth
    b. striated
    c. cardiac
    d. uninucleated
    e. involuntary

Answer:

28. Intercalated disks are found in which type of muscle?

    a. smooth
    b. striated
    c. cardiac
    d. multinucleated
    e. voluntary

Answer:

29. In the nerve cell, stimuli are received by the

    a. neuroglia
    b. axon
    c. dendrite
    d. cell body
    e. myelin

Answer:

30. The supporting cells of the nervous system are the

    a. neuroglia
    b. axon
    c. dendrite
    d. cell body
    e. myelin

Answer:

31. An example of dense connective tissue with an irregular arrangement of fibers is a(n)

    a. aponeurosis
    b. muscle sheath
    c. tendon
    d. ligament
    e. fibroblast

Answer:

32. Bone stores the mineral salts calcium and

    a. adenosine
    b. potassium
    c. phosphorus
    d. chloride
    e. sodium

Answer:

CHAPTER 6

The Integumentary System

OBJECTIVES

After studying this chapter, you should be able to:

1. Name the layers of the epidermis.
2. Define keratinization.
3. Explain why there are skin color differences among people.
4. Describe the anatomic parts of a hair.
5. Compare the two kinds of glands in the skin based on structure and secretion.
6. Explain why sweating is important to survival.
7. Explain how the skin helps regulate body temperature.
8. Name the functions of the skin.

ACTIVITIES

A. Completion

Fill in the blank spaces with the correct term.

1. One of the ways the skin helps regulate body temperature is through the evaporation of ___.
2. The epidermis is a layer of ___ tissue.
3. The second layer is the ___.
4. The dermis is a layer of ___ tissue.

NAME: _____   DATE: _____

5. The epidermis is composed of ___, ___, and ___ cells.

6. The skin is thickest on the ___ of the hands and the ___ of the feet.

7. As cells move up from the basement membrane, they eventually ___.

8. The protein material of hair and nails is ___.

9. There are ___ layers of the epidermis.

10. Dead cells converted to protein make up the ___ ___.

11. A callus on the foot is called a(n) ___.

12. Cells lose their nuclei and become compact and brittle in the ___.

13. The stratum spinosum contain cells that are ___ in structure.

14. Cells of the epidermis that are capable of dividing are found in the ___ ___.

15. Those cells responsible for skin color are ___.

16. Racial variation in skin color is determined by ___.

17. An absence of melanin produces a condition called ___.

18. True skin is the ___.

19. A specialist concerned with inflammatory responses of the skin and reactions of the immune system is a(n) ___.

20. Besides mammary glands, ___ is a main characteristic of mammals.

21. A bluish tinge to the skin is called ___.

22. Goose bumps are caused by the ___ ___ muscle.

23. Hair growth begins in the ___ ___.

24. A nail will grow from the ___ ___.

25. The eponychium is the ___.

26. ___ is the oily substance responsible for lubrication of the skin and is a product of the ___ ___.

27. The hands and feet are the site of many ___ ___.

28. Sweating causes odor because of ___ activity.

29. Sensations recorded by the skin are ___ and ___.

30. Inhibition of water loss by the skin is due to its ___ content.

31. A common chronic skin disorder is ___.

32. Herpes simplex causes ___ ___.

33. The varicella (chickenpox) virus is responsible for ___.

34. Sweat glands are activated by ___.

35. A patchy skin disease is ___.

36. A vaccine is available for children 12 months or older to prevent ___, caused by the virus varicella-zoster.

37. Impetigo is caused by the bacterium ___ ___.

38. The dermis is also known as the ___.

B. Matching

Match the term on the right with the definition on the left.

_____ 39. skin modifications   a. epidermis

_____ 40. epidermal cellular links   b. shaft

_____ 41. clear layer   c. sweat

_____ 42. varies skin pigmentation   d. keratin

_____ 43. affected by first-degree burns   e. appendages

_____ 44. subcutaneous layer   f. warts

_____ 45. hair's principal portion   g. nail body

_____ 46. hair's visible portion   h. desmosomes

_____ 47. hair texture   i. hypodermis

_____ 48. visible nail   j. melanin

_____ 49. oily gland   k. melanoma

_____ 50. salty liquid secretion   l. stratum lucidum

_____ 51. skin function   m. cortex

_____ 52. skin cancer   n. thermoregulation

_____ 53. human *Papillomavirus*   o. sebaceous

C. Key Terms

Use the text to look up the following terms. Write the definition or explanation.

54. Albinism:

_____

_____

55. Arrector pili muscle:

_____

_____

56. Basal cell carcinoma:

_____

_____

57. Callus:

_____

_____

58. Cold sores:

_____

_____

59. Corium:

_____

_____

60. Corns:

_____

_____

61. Cortex:

_____

_____

62. Cuticle:

_____

_____

63. Cyanosis:

_____

_____

64. Dermis:

_____

_____

65. Desmosome:

_____

_____

66. Epidermis:

_____

_____

67. First-degree burns:

_____

_____

68. Full-thickness burns:

_____

_____

69. Hair:

_____

_____

70. Hair follicle:

_____

_____

71. Hypodermis:

_____

_____

72. Keratin:

_____

_____

73. Keratinization:

_____

_____

74. Lunula:

_____

_____

75. Malignant melanoma:

_____

_____

76. Medulla:

_____

_____

77. Melanocytes:

_____

_____

78. Melanin:

_____

_____

79. Nail bed:

_____

_____

80. Nail body:

_____

_____

81. Nail root:

_____

_____

82. Papillary portion:

_____

_____

83. Partial-thickness burns:

_____

_____

84. Reticular portion:

_____

_____

85. Root:

_____

_____

86. Sebaceous glands:

_____

_____

87. Sebum:

_____

_____

88. Second-degree burns:

_____

_____

89. Shaft:

_____

_____

90. Squamous cell carcinoma:

_____

_____

91. Strata:

_____

_____

92. Stratum basale:

_____

_____

93. Stratum corneum:

_____

_____

94. Stratum germinativum:

_____

_____

95. Stratum granulosum:

_____

_____

96. Stratum lucidum:

_____

_____

97. Stratum spinosum:

_____

_____

98. Sweat glands:

_____

_____

99. Third-degree burns:

_____

_____

D. Labeling Exercise

100. Label the parts of the skin as indicated in Figure 6-1.

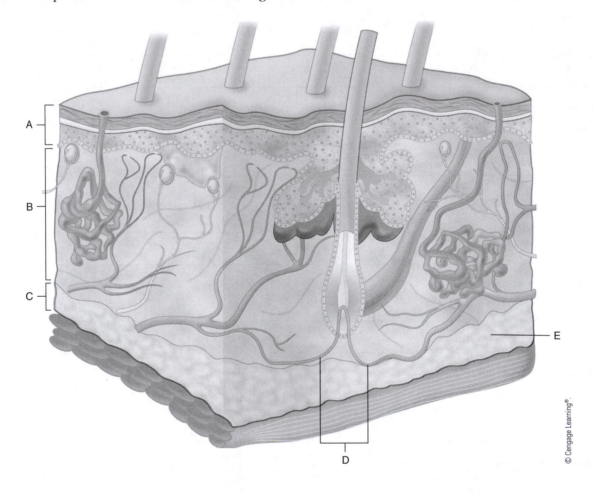

Figure 6-1

A. _____   D. _____

B. _____   E. _____

C. _____

101. Label the parts of the hair as indicated in Figure 6-2.

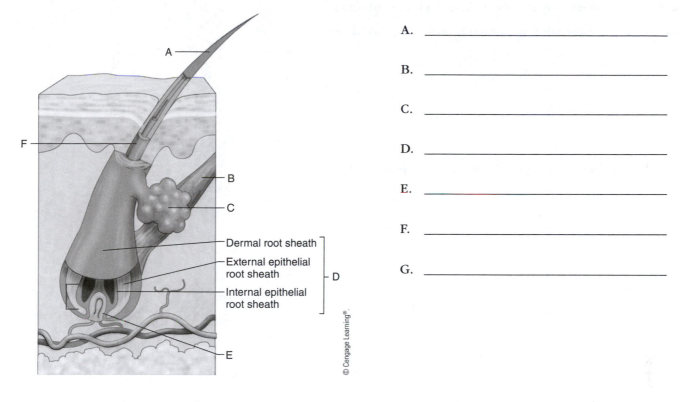

A. _____

B. _____

C. _____

D. _____

E. _____

F. _____

G. _____

Figure 6-2

E. Coloring Exercise

102. Using Figure 6-3, color the nail bed red, the lunula brown, and the nail blue.

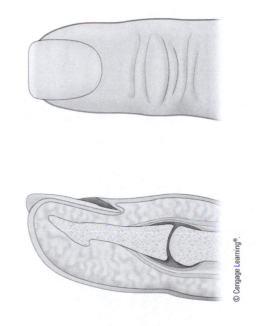

Figure 6-3

F. Critical Thinking

Answer the following questions in complete sentences.

103. How does the stratum corneum protect against disease?

104. Why is the stratum germinativum so important?

105. Why are third-degree burns so traumatic?

106. Why is the dermis called the true skin?

107. Why would deep tissue trauma cause hair loss?

108. If a nail is completely torn out, why does it grow back?

109. Explain why adolescents experience more acne than adults.

110. Is the sweat gland an exocrine or endocrine gland?

111. Why are sports drinks so important to athletes?

112. How can impetigo cause other diseases?

113. Is ringworm a correct term for the disease?

114. What changes occur in the integumentary system as the body ages?

G. Crossword Puzzle

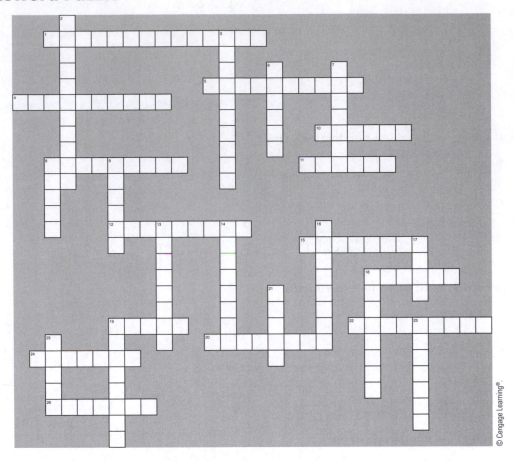

© Cengage Learning®.

Complete the crossword puzzle using the following clues.

ACROSS

1. Skin cell process
4. Subcutaneous tissue
5. Cellular links
8. Oily glands
10. Distinctive layers
11. White crescent of the nail
12. Outer layer of skin
15. Fungi-caused skin disease
18. Thickened skin area
19. Visible part of hair
20. Bacteria-caused skin disease
22. System that secretes hormones
24. Skin pigmentation
26. Middle part of hair

DOWN

2. Produces skin color
3. Means a covering
6. True skin
7. Protein material
8. Cools skin
9. Principal portion of hair
13. Shedding scalp cells
14. Absence of skin color
16. Irregular patches of skin pigmentation
17. Groupings of melanocytes
18. Bluish skin discoloration
19. Disease caused by the chickenpox virus
21. Caused by human *Papillomavirus*
23. Eponychium
25. Oil for skin lubrication

CASE STUDY

Deniz, a 52-year-old woman, is hospitalized following the removal of a cancerous section of her colon. Deniz is having difficulty coping with her situation, and she repeatedly states that she feels very "stressed out and doesn't know how she will ever recover." During the night, Deniz tells her health care provider she is experiencing severe pain beneath her left arm and across the left side of her back. The health care provider examines Deniz and finds vesicular skin eruptions across the left side of her back that extend beneath her left arm.

QUESTIONS

1. What condition might Deniz have suddenly developed?

2. What is the cause of this condition?

3. Deniz's medical history should document that she had which childhood infection?

4. How is this condition treated?

CHAPTER QUIZ

1. A bony prominence on the foot receiving excess friction may develop a

   a. ringworm infection
   b. wart
   c. blackhead

   d. corn
   e. none of the above

Answer:

2. Albinism is caused by a lack of

   a. desmosome
   b. osteocytes
   c. melanocytes

   d. mast cells
   e. none of the above

Answer:

3. Excessive production of sebum may cause

   a. psoriasis
   b. callus
   c. corns

   d. shingles
   e. none of the above

Answer:

4. Keratinized cells contain no

   a. nucleus
   b. cell wall
   c. fluid

   d. cell membrane
   e. none of the above

Answer:

5. Flexibility, entirety, and whole continuous structure are qualities of the skin due to

   a. a callus
   b. desmosomes
   c. melanocytes

   d. osteocytes
   e. corns

Answer:

6. The layer of the epidermis in which mitosis takes place is the stratum

   a. spinosum
   b. granulosum
   c. germinativum

   d. corneum
   e. lucidum

Answer:

7. A lipid covering of cells is found in the stratum

   a. spinosum
   b. granulosum
   c. germinativum

   d. corneum
   e. lucidum

Answer:

8. Cells of the stratum corneum contain as many as

   a. 10 layers
   b. 5 layers
   c. 20 layers

   d. 25 layers
   e. none of the above

Answer:

9. Stratum basale is found in the stratum

   a. spinosum
   b. granulosum
   c. germinativum

   d. corneum
   e. lucidum

Answer:

10. Racial color differences are a result of variation in quantity of

   a. astrocytes
   b. desmosome
   c. melanocytes

   d. karyocytes
   e. none of the above

Answer:

11. True skin contains which of the following?

   a. papillary portion
   b. hypodermis
   c. areolar tissue

   d. adipose tissue
   e. none of the above

Answer:

12. A bluish tinge of the skin is called

    a. psoriasis
    b. cyanosis
    c. shingles
    d. ringworm
    e. none of the above

Answer:

13. Besides hair, another main characteristic of mammals is

    a. sweat glands
    b. ceruminous glands
    c. mammary glands
    d. adrenal glands
    e. none of the above

Answer:

14. Hair covers all of the body EXCEPT the

    a. arms
    b. legs
    c. face
    d. palms of the hands
    e. none of the above

Answer:

15. Arrector pili muscles engage when we get

    a. a chill
    b. psoriasis
    c. a papillomavirus
    d. shingles
    e. cold sores

Answer:

16. Texture of hair is a result of

    a. melanocytes
    b. astrocytes
    c. desmosomes
    d. melanin
    e. keratin

Answer:

17. A white crescent located at the proximal end of the nail is the

    a. nail bed
    b. lunula
    c. cuticle
    d. root
    e. none of the above

Answer:

18. Another name for the eponychium is

    a. cuticle
    b. nail body
    c. nail bed
    d. lunula
    e. nail root

Answer:

19. Shiny hair is a result of

    a. melanocytes
    b. sebum
    c. sweat
    d. callus
    e. cerumen

Answer:

20. Sebaceous secretion is controlled by the

    a. exocrine system
    b. lymphatic system
    c. endocrine system

    d. circulatory system
    e. none of the above

Answer:

21. Besides fatty oils, blackheads are produced in the presence of

    a. water
    b. heat
    c. cold

    d. air
    e. none of the above

Answer:

22. Sweat odor is caused by

    a. melanocytes
    b. astrocytes
    c. desmosomes

    d. bacteria
    e. yeast

Answer:

23. External environmental changes are registered by receptor sites; these changes are

    a. wet and dry
    b. temperature and moisture
    c. pressure and moisture

    d. temperature and pressure
    e. none of the above

Answer:

24. Which of the following are NOT protective functions?

    a. sunlight
    b. bacteria
    c. some chemical agents

    d. water loss
    e. organic pesticides

Answer:

25. Temperature regulation is critical due to excessive heat affecting

    a. enzymes
    b. blood
    c. urea

    d. sugar
    e. water

Answer:

26. A condition characterized by baldness that is influenced by genetic factors, hormones, malnutrition, diabetes, drug interactions, and/or chemotherapy is

    a. molds
    b. alopecia
    c. psoriasis

    d. vitiligo
    e. impetigo

Answer:

27. The skin is involved in the production of

    a. ATP
    b. phosphate
    c. calcium

    d. vitamin D
    e. none of the above

Answer:

28. The most dangerous type of skin cancer is

    a. malignant melanoma
    b. basal cell carcinoma
    c. squamous cell carcinoma
    d. keratinized carcinoma
    e. none of the above

Answer:

29. A children's disease that can cause a related disease in adults is

    a. ringworm
    b. chickenpox
    c. psoriasis
    d. impetigo
    e. none of the above

Answer:

30. The type I herpes simplex virus causes

    a. warts
    b. impetigo
    c. shingles
    d. cold sores
    e. psoriasis

Answer:

31. The nail is a modification of

    a. sebaceous glands
    b. muscle cells
    c. hair cells
    d. dermal cells
    e. epidermal cells

Answer:

32. Which of the following transmit information from receptor sites in the skin to the brain and spinal cord?

    a. sensory neurons
    b. sweat glands
    c. chemical agents
    d. melanocytes
    e. viruses

Answer:

33. Keratinization produces distinct layers of the epidermis called

    a. strata
    b. neurons
    c. desmosomes
    d. integuments
    e. melanocytes

Answer:

CHAPTER 7

The Skeletal System

OBJECTIVES

After studying this chapter, you should be able to:

1. Name the functions of the skeletal system.

2. Name the two types of ossification.

3. Describe why diet can affect bone development in children and bone maintenance in older adults.

4. Describe the histology of compact bone.

5. Define and give examples of bone markings.

6. Name the cranial and facial bones.

7. Name the bones of the axial and appendicular skeleton.

ACTIVITIES

A. Completion

Fill in the blank spaces with the correct term.

1. The five functions of the skeletal system include ___, ___, ___, ___, and ___ ___.

2. Osteoblasts invade ___ and begin the process of ossification.

3. The ___ is a fibrovascular membrane that covers bone; the ___ is the membrane that lines the medullary cavity.

4. Bone remodeling is made possible by ___ and ___.

5. The process of ossification can be either ___ or ___.

NAME: _____   DATE: _____

6. Correct calcium ion concentration in blood and bone is maintained by ___ and ___.

7. ___ bone is dense and strong, whereas ___ bone is spongy.

8. An osteon, also called the ___ ___, allows for the effective metabolism of bone cells.

9. The spaces within cancellous bone contain ___ ___ ___, which is responsible for hematopoiesis.

10. Long bones consist of a(n) ___, ___, and a(n) ___.

11. ___ bones are enclosed in a tendon and fascial tissue.

12. An obvious bony prominence is called a(n) ___.

13. A depression or cavity in or on a bone is called a(n) ___.

14. The skeleton is divided into two main parts, the ___ and the ___.

15. The ___ bone is a single bone that forms the posterior base of the cranium.

16. The anchor bone for the cranium is the ___ ___ ___.

17. The freely movable bone of the face is the ___ ___.

18. The spinal cord passes through a space called the ___ ___.

19. The largest and strongest vertebrae are those of the ___ section of the spine.

20. ___ are the bones of the fingers and toes.

21. ___ is the manufacture of red blood cells.

22. The turbinates are also called the nasal ___ bones.

23. A black eye is also known as a(n) ___ ecchymosis or bruise.

B. Matching

Match the term on the right with the definition on the left.

_____ 24. result of abnormal endochondral ossification at the epiphyseal plate of long bones
                                                  a. osteoporosis

_____ 25. lateral curvature of the spine
                                                  b. lordosis

_____ 26. the laminae of the posterior vertebral arch do not unite at the midline
                                                  c. giantism

_____ 27. disorder characterized by disease in bone mass with increased susceptibility to fractures
                                                  d. axis

_____ 28. rupture of fibrocartilage surrounding an intervertebral disk
                                                  e. kyphosis

_____ 29. irregular thickening and softening of the bones with excessive bone destruction
                                                  f. scoliosis

_____ 30. swayback
                                                  g. false ribs

_____ 31. strongest portion of the hip bone
                                                  h. spina bifida

_____ 32. accentuated curvature of the spine in the upper thoracic region
                                                  i. herniated disk

_____ 33. second vertebra
                                                  j. incus

_____ 34. direct articulation with the sternum
                                                  k. patella

_____ 35. indirect articulation with the sternum
                                                  l. carpals

_____ 36. do not attach anteriorly

_____ 37. bones of the wrist

_____ 38. anvil

_____ 39. kneecap

_____ 40. give rise to osteoblasts

_____ 41. immovable joint line of the cranium

_____ 42. tie bone to bones

_____ 43. tongue attached to it

m. ischium

n. true ribs

o. hyoid

p. osteoprogenitor

q. Paget's disease

r. floating ribs

s. suture

t. ligaments

C. Key Terms

Use the text to look up the following terms. Write the definition or explanation.

44. Acetabulum:

_____

_____

45. Acromegaly:

_____

_____

46. Acromial process:

_____

_____

47. Alveolus:

_____

_____

48. Atlas:

_____

_____

49. Auditory ossicles:

_____

_____

50. Axis:

_____

_____

51. Calcaneus:

_____

_____

52. Canaliculi:

_____

_____

53. Cancellous or spongy bone:

_____

_____

54. Capitate:

_____

_____

55. Carpals:

_____

_____

56. Cartilage:

_____

_____

57. Cervical vertebrae:

_____

_____

58. Clavicle:

_____

_____

59. Coccygeal vertebrae/coccyx:

_____

_____

60. Compact or dense bone:

_____

_____

61. Condyle:

_____

_____

62. Coracoid process:

_____

_____

63. Coronal suture:

_____

_____

64. Costae:

_____

_____

65. Crest:

_____

_____

66. Cuboid:

_____

_____

67. Cuneiforms:

_____

_____

68. Diaphysis:

_____

_____

69. Endochondral ossification:

_____

_____

70. Endosteum:

_____

_____

71. Epiphyseal line:

_____

_____

72. Epiphysis:

_____

_____

73. Ethmoid bone:

_____

_____

74. External occipital crest:

_____

_____

75. External occipital protuberance:

_____

_____

76. Femur:

_____

_____

77. Fibula:

_____

_____

78. Fontanelle:

_____

_____

79. Foramen:

_____

_____

80. Foramen magnum:

_____

_____

81. Fossae:

_____

_____

82. Fracture:

_____

_____

83. Frontal bone:

_____

_____

84. Gladiolus:

_____

_____

85. Glenoid fossa:

_____

_____

86. Hamate:

_____

_____

87. Haversian (system):

_____

_____

88. Head:

_____

_____

89. Hematopoiesis:

_____

_____

90. Humerus:

_____

_____

91. Hyoid bone:

_____

_____

92. Ilium:

_____

_____

93. Incus:

_____

_____

94. Intramembranous ossification:

_____

_____

95. Ischium:

_____

_____

96. Kyphosis:

_____

_____

97. Lacrimal bones:

_____

_____

98. Lacunae:

_____

_____

99. Lamella:

_____

_____

100. Lambdoid suture:

_____

_____

101. Ligaments:

_____

_____

102. Line:

_____

_____

103. Lordosis:

_____

_____

104. Lumbar vertebrae:

_____

_____

105. Lunate:

_____

_____

106. Malleus:

_____

_____

107. Mandible bone:

_____

_____

108. Manubrium:

_____

_____

109. Mastoid portion of temporal bone:

_____

_____

110. Maxillary bones:

_____

_____

111. Meatus:

_____

_____

112. Medullary cavity:

_____

_____

113. Metacarpal bones:

_____

_____

114. Metaphysis:

_____

_____

115. Metatarsals:

_____

_____

116. Nasal bones:

_____

_____

117. Navicular/scaphoid:

_____

_____

118. Neck:

_____

_____

119. Obturator foramen:

_____

_____

120. Occipital bone:

_____

_____

121. Occipital condyle:

_____

_____

122. Olecranon process:

_____

_____

123. Orbital margin:

_____

_____

124. Ossification:

_____

_____

125. Osteoblasts:

_____

_____

126. Osteoclasts:

_____

_____

127. Osteomalacia:

_____

_____

128. Osteon:

_____

_____

129. Osteoprogenitor cell:

_____

_____

130. Palatine bones:

_____

_____

131. Parietal bones:

_____

_____

132. Patella:

_____

_____

133. Pelvic girdle:

_____

_____

134. Periosteum:

_____

_____

135. Petrous part of temporal bone:

_____

_____

136. Phalanges:

_____

_____

137. Phalanx:

_____

_____

138. Pisiform:

_____

_____

139. Processes:

_____

_____

140. Pubis:

_____

_____

141. Radius:

_____

_____

142. Red bone marrow:

_____

_____

143. Sacral vertebrae/sacrum:

_____

_____

144. Sagittal suture:

_____

_____

145. Scaphoid/navicular:

_____

_____

146. Scapula:

_____

_____

147. Scoliosis:

_____

_____

148. Sesamoid bones:

_____

_____

149. Sinus/antrum:

_____

_____

150. Sinusitis:

_____

_____

151. Sphenoid bones:

_____

_____

152. Spine:

_____

_____

153. Squamous portion of temporal bone:

_____

_____

154. Stapes:

_____

_____

155. Sternum:

_____

_____

156. Sulcus/groove:

_____

_____

157. Supraorbital ridge:

_____

_____

158. Suture:

_____

_____

159. Talus:

_____

_____

160. Tarsal bones:

_____

_____

161. Temporal bones:

_____

_____

162. Tendons:

_____

_____

163. Thoracic vertebrae:

_____

_____

164. Tibia:

_____

_____

165. Trabeculae:

_____

_____

166. Trapezium:

_____

_____

167. Trapezoid:

_____

_____

168. Triquetral:

_____

_____

169. Trochanter:

_____

_____

170. Trochlea:

_____

_____

171. Tubercle:

_____

_____

172. Turbinates or nasal conchae bones:

_____

_____

173. Tympanic plate:

_____

_____

174. Ulna:

_____

_____

175. Volkmann's/perforating canals:

_____

_____

176. Vomer (bone):

_____

_____

177. Wormian/sutural bones:

_____

_____

178. Xiphoid:

_____

_____

179. Yellow bone marrow:

_____

_____

180. Zygomatic (bones):

_____

_____

D. Labeling Exercise

181. Label the bones of the skeletal system as indicated in Figure 7-1.

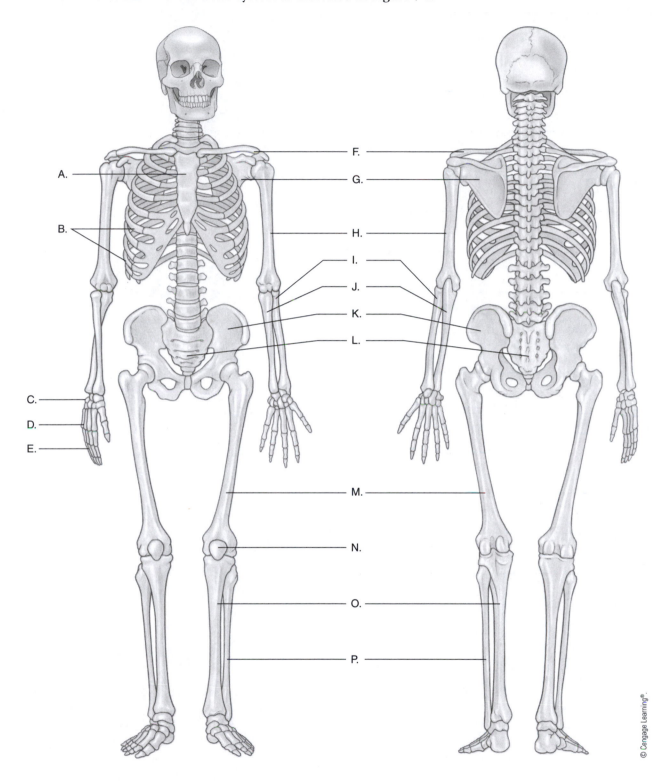

Figure 7-1

A. _____

B. _____

C. _____

D. _____

E. _____

F. _____

G. _____

H. _____

I. _____

J. _____

K. _____

L. _____

M. _____

N. _____

O. _____

P. _____

182. **Label the parts of the spinal column as indicated in Figure 7-2.**

A. C₁ _____

B. C₂ _____

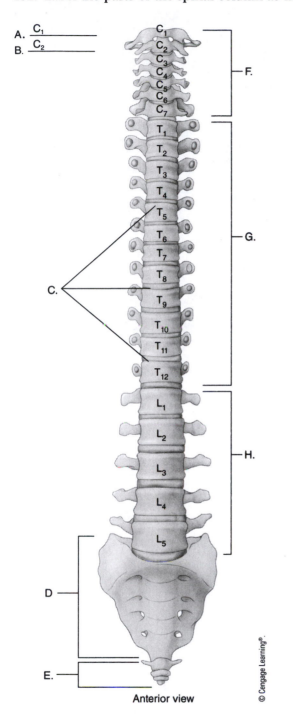

Anterior view

Figure 7-2

A. _____

B. _____

C. _____

D. _____

E. _____

F. _____

G. _____

H. _____

183. Label the bones of the thoracic cage as indicated in Figure 7-3.

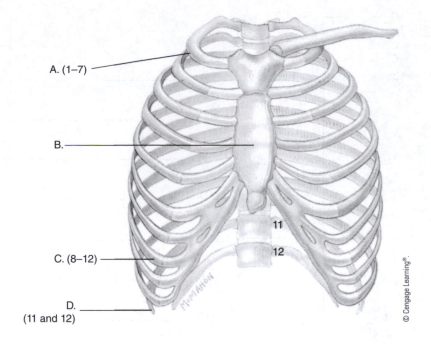

A. (1–7)

B.

C. (8–12)

11

12

D.
(11 and 12)

© Cengage Learning®.

Figure 7-3

A. _____

B. _____

C. _____

D. _____

184. Label the bones of the hand and wrist as indicated in Figure 7-4.

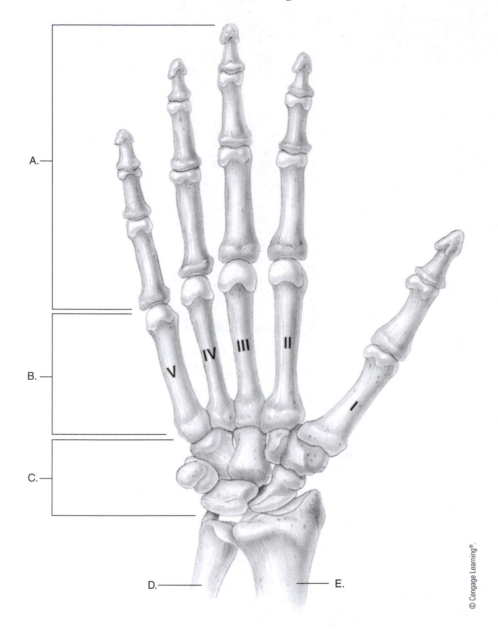

Figure 7-4

A. _____

B. _____

C. _____

D. _____

E. _____

185. Label the bones of the foot as indicated in Figure 7-5.

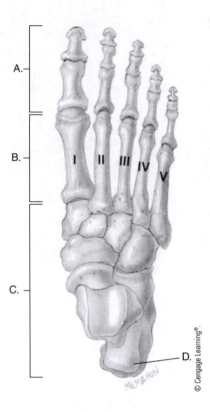

Figure 7-5

A. _____

B. _____

C. _____

D. _____

E. Coloring Exercise

186. Using Figure 7-6, color the skull blue, the axial skeleton green, and the appendicular skeleton red.

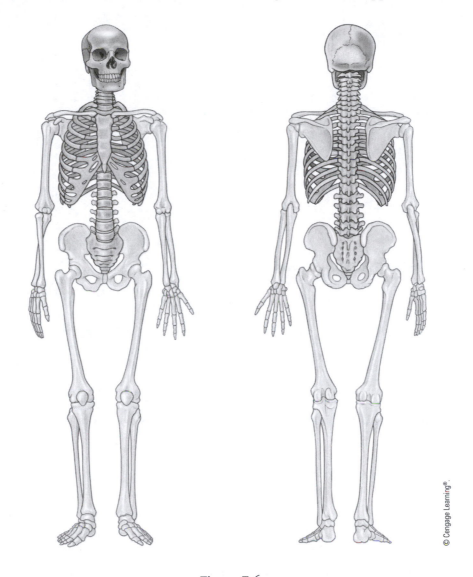

Figure 7-6

F. Critical Thinking

Answer the following questions in complete sentences.

187. Why is the calcaneus a large strong bone?

188. Differentiate osteoblast, osteoclast, and osteoprogenitor cell.

189. How does the body maintain proper calcium balance?

190. Differentiate red and yellow bone marrow.

191. What defect results from fusion failure of the maxillary bones? Why would it affect speech?

192. Why are the 11th and 12th pairs of ribs called "floating ribs"?

193. The glenoid fossa is similar to what structure of the hip?

194. Why is rickets a common disease in many third world countries?

195. Differentiate between tendon and ligament.

196. Explain how aging affects bone and its supporting tissues.

197. Identify the skeletal system career option that would best fit your interests and explain why.

198. Briefly explain the difference among an orthotist, an orthopedist, and a prosthetist.

199. Describe what a Doctor of Chiropractic, or chiropractor, does and the training required to become one.

G. Crossword Puzzle

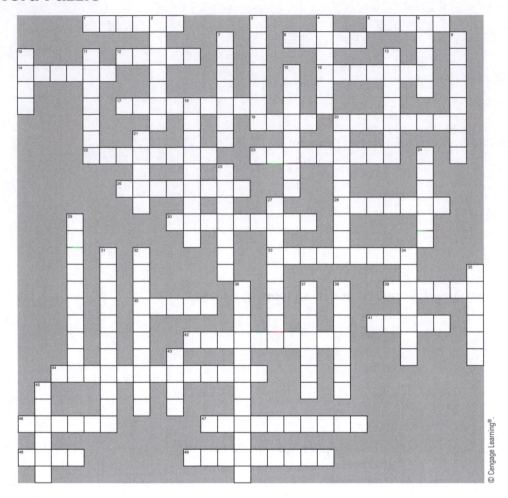

Complete the crossword puzzle using the following clues.

ACROSS

1. Narrow junction between two bones
5. Sharp, slender projection
8. Bone supporting the tongue
12. Ear bone referred to as the anvil
14. Five unfused vertebrae in the lower back
16. Shoulder blade
17. Mature osteoblast
19. Connects the head to the rest of a long bone
20. 12 vertebrae that connect with the ribs
22. Small rounded bone
23. Perforating canals
26. Bones that make up part of the orbit of the inner angle of the eye
28. Forms the dense, outer layer of bone

DOWN

2. Disease caused by lack of vitamin D
3. Opening in bone for nerve or blood vessel, etc.
4. Bone depressions
6. Bones forming the bridge of the nose
7. Knuckle-like prominence at an articulation point
9. Small, rounded process
10. Bone type that protects vital body parts
11. Ear bone referred to as the hammer
13. Longest bone of the upper arm
15. Pulley-shaped process
18. Single bone forming the back of the cranium
20. Meshwork of interconnecting bone sections
21. Zygomatic bone
24. Furrow or groove

30. Part of the sternum resembling the handle of a sword

33. Finger bones

39. Long, tubelike passage

40. Narrow ridge of bone

41. Cavity within a bone

42. Fibrovascular membrane covering a bone

44. Making blood cells

46. Shorter bone of the forearm

47. Flared portion at the ends of a long bone

48. Terminal enlargement of a bone

49. Lines the medullary cavity of long bones

25. Tiny cavities between lamellae

27. Shaft of long bone

29. Soft spot on a baby's head

31. Cells responsible for reabsorption of bone

32. Spongy bone

34. Breastbone

35. Haversian canal

36. Formation of bone by osteoblasts

37. Ring of bone around the haversian canal

38. Bone supporting the nasal cavity structure

43. Bone whose length exceeds its width

45. Ear bone referred to as the stirrup

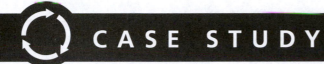

CASE STUDY

Aayshah, a 13-year-old girl, is being evaluated by her health care provider. Aayshah, who has an abnormal curvature of her spine in the thoracic region, was born with one leg slightly shorter than the other. The health care provider determines that the curvature is progressing in severity, and she refers Aayshah to an orthotist for treatment.

QUESTIONS

1. For what skeletal problem is Aayshah being treated?

2. What are the major causes of this condition?

3. What is the role of an orthotist in treating individuals with orthopedic disorders?

CHAPTER QUIZ

1. Which of the following is NOT a function of the skeletal system?

   a. support
   b. protection
   c. nutrient absorption
   d. movement
   e. storage of mineral salts

   Answer:

2. Longitudinal growth of bone continues until approximately what age in boys?

   a. 15
   b. 13
   c. 14

   d. 21
   e. 16

Answer:

3. Undifferentiated bone cells are called

   a. osteoclasts
   b. osteoprogenitors
   c. osteoblasts

   d. osteons
   e. osteocytes

Answer:

4. The skeletal system is most closely associated with which system?

   a. respiratory
   b. digestive
   c. excretory

   d. muscular
   e. lymphatic

Answer:

5. The hormones responsible for proper calcium balance in the body are

   a. calcitonin/potassium
   b. thyroxine/calcitonin
   c. renin/parathormone

   d. parathormone/calcitonin
   e. progesterone/epinephrine

Answer:

6. Osteomalacia in adults is known as what disease in children?

   a. measles
   b. spina bifida
   c. Paget's disease

   d. rickets
   e. Graves disease

Answer:

7. Hematopoiesis takes place in which type of bone?

   a. compact
   b. flat
   c. hard

   d. short
   e. cancellous

Answer:

8. The haversian system is necessary for

   a. maintaining calcium balance
   b. hematopoiesis
   c. protection of soft tissue

   d. ossification
   e. effective metabolism of bone cells

Answer:

9. Blood cells in all stages of development are found in

   a. lacunae
   b. canaliculi
   c. yellow marrow

   d. red marrow
   e. Volkmann's canals

Answer:

10. Bones can be divided into how many categories based on shape?

    a. 5
    b. 7
    c. 2
    d. 10
    e. 3

Answer:

11. Long bones have a shaft called a(n)

    a. epiphysis
    b. diaphysis
    c. metaphysis
    d. osteon
    e. medullary

Answer:

12. The medullary shaft is filled with

    a. blood
    b. yellow marrow
    c. red marrow
    d. cartilage
    e. trabeculae

Answer:

13. Examples of flat bones are

    a. wrist/ankle
    b. ribs/scapula
    c. tibia/fibula
    d. carpal/tarsal
    e. vertebrae/auditory ossicles

Answer:

14. A sesamoid bone is the

    a. patella
    b. sternum
    c. clavicle
    d. phalanges
    e. mandible

Answer:

15. Which of the following is NOT a process?

    a. meatus
    b. condyle
    c. tubercle
    d. crest
    e. trochlea

Answer:

16. Which of the following is NOT a fossa?

    a. suture
    b. sinus
    c. trochanter
    d. sulcus
    e. foramen

Answer:

17. Which two bones form the upper sides and roof of the cranium?

    a. occipital
    b. frontal
    c. parietal
    d. temporal
    e. sphenoid

Answer:

18. The cheekbones are which bones?

    a. nasal
    b. palatine
    c. malar

    d. lacrimal
    e. turbinates

Answer:

19. Bones act as storage areas for mineral salts and

    a. muscle tissue
    b. blood
    c. fats

    d. lymph
    e. waste

Answer:

20. Which bone of the axial skeleton has no articulation with other bones?

    a. vomer
    b. temporal
    c. hyoid

    d. palatine
    e. occipital

Answer:

21. There are how many sections of the spine?

    a. 4
    b. 15
    c. 7

    d. 5
    e. 10

Answer:

22. The two sections of the spine that consist of fused bones are the

    a. cervical/coccygeal
    b. thoracic/sacrum
    c. lumbar/cervical

    d. sacrum/lumbar
    e. coccygeal/sacrum

Answer:

23. Abnormal curvature of the spine in the lumbar region is known as swayback or

    a. kyphosis
    b. rickets
    c. osteoporosis

    d. Paget's disease
    e. lordosis

Answer:

24. The manubrium articulates with the

    a. scapula
    b. axis
    c. sacrum

    d. acromion process
    e. clavicle

Answer:

25. The lower five pairs of ribs are called

    a. true ribs
    b. floating ribs
    c. false ribs

    d. costal ribs
    e. paired ribs

Answer:

26. Two bony projections of the scapula are called the

    a. acromial processes
    b. glenoid processes
    c. coracoid processes

    d. acetabulum
    e. spinous processes

Answer:

27. The longer bone of the forearm is the

    a. humerus
    b. radius
    c. ulna

    d. scaphoid
    e. carpal

Answer:

28. The coxal bones make up the

    a. pubis
    b. ischium
    c. ilium

    d. acetabulum
    e. pelvic girdle

Answer:

29. The longest and heaviest bone of the body is the

    a. ilium
    b. tibia
    c. humerus

    d. patella
    e. femur

Answer:

30. The shinbone is the

    a. tibia
    b. fibula
    c. calcaneus

    d. patella
    e. femur

Answer:

31. Which of the foot bones is the largest?

    a. cuboid
    b. phalanges
    c. calcaneus

    d. navicular
    e. talus

Answer:

32. Decreased height of the longitudinal arches is known as

    a. rickets
    b. Graves disease
    c. kyphosis

    d. tinea pedis
    e. pes planus

Answer:

33. Which of the following is NOT a bone of the axial skeleton?

    a. sternum
    b. occipital
    c. xiphoid

    d. radius
    e. coccyx

Answer:

34. Which of the following is NOT a bone of the appendicular skeleton?

     a. ulna   d. patella
     b. ribs   e. calcaneus
     c. femur

Answer:

35. Which of the following attaches bone to bone?

     a. tendons   d. muscle
     b. aponeurosis   e. none of the above
     c. ligament

Answer:

36. The metaphysis consists mainly of

     a. tendons   d. muscle
     b. spongy bone   e. ligaments
     c. compact bone

Answer:

37. What is the name for the two deep cavities in the upper portion of the face that protect the eyes?

     a. orbits   d. vomers
     b. aponeuroses   e. palatines
     c. metaphyses

Answer:

38. During labor and birth, epidural anesthetics are commonly given in

     a. the shoulders   d. the lumbar region
     b. the sternum   e. the cervical region
     c. the ribs

Answer:

The Articular System

OBJECTIVES

After studying this chapter, you should be able to:

1. Name and describe the three types of joints.

2. Name the two types of synarthroses joints.

3. Name examples of the two types of amphiarthroses joints.

4. Name and give examples of the six types of diarthroses or synovial joints.

5. Describe the capsular nature of a synovial joint.

6. Describe the three types of bursae.

7. Name some of the disorders of joints.

8. Describe the possible movements at synovial joints.

ACTIVITIES

A. Completion

Fill in the blank spaces with the correct term.

1. A union between two or more bones is a(n) ___.

2. Joints are classified by ___ and ___.

3. Skull joints are called ___.

4. Besides sutures, there are two other types of synarthroses; they are ___ and ___.

5. Those joints allowing only slight movement are ___.

NAME: _____   DATE: _____

6. A joint in which two bony surfaces are connected by hyaline cartilage is a(n) ___.

7. Synovial joints are also called ___.

8. Synovial joints are characterized by the presence of a(n) ___ and a(n) ___.

9. A diarthrosis joint provides a smooth gliding surface because of ___.

10. A buffer between two weight-bearing bones is provided by ___.

11. The joint providing the greatest range of motion in the body is found in the ___.

12. Functions of the synovial joints include ___, ___, and ___.

13. A decrease in the angle of a joint is denoted as ___.

14. If a joint is forced beyond its normal range of extension, it is ___.

15. Movement of a limb away from the midline of the body is ___.

16. Moving a limb in a direction that causes the bone to describe a cone is ___.

17. ___ is a movement placing the palm in an anterior position.

18. Moving the palm of the hand so that it faces down is called ___.

19. Move the body forward for ___ and backward for ___.

20. ___ is raising the body.

21. Only primates can perform the movement called ___.

22. A ball-and-socket joint will have a ball-shaped head fitting into a(n) ___ ___.

23. In the joint of the hip, the ball-shaped head of the femur fits into the ___.

24. An example of a hinge joint is the ___.

25. A condyloid joint is also known as a(n) ___ joint.

26. The thumb is an example of a(n) ___ joint.

27. Gliding joints are found in the ___.

28. Closed sacs with a synovial lining are ___.

29. Inflammation of a joint is called ___.

30. Degenerative joint disease is sometimes known as ___.

31. ___ is an inflammation of the tissues of the gum.

32. A sprain occurs when a twisting or turning action tears ___.

33. Supination and ___ refer to the movement of the forearm and hand.

B. Matching

Match the term on the right with the definition on the left.

_____ 34. accumulation of uric acid crystals   a. depression

_____ 35. rheumatism   b. pivot joint

_____ 36. connective tissue disorder   c. extension

_____ 37. inflammation of synovial bursa   d. gout

_____ 38. bacterial infection   e. primary fibrositis

_____ 39. one tendon overlies another

_____ 40. subfascial bursae

_____ 41. example, atlas vertebra

_____ 42. lowering part of the body

_____ 43. move the sole outward

_____ 44. increase joint angle

_____ 45. move around the central axis

_____ 46. pushing the foot up

_____ 47. move the limb toward the midline

_____ 48. reinforce a joint capsule

f. adduction

g. ligaments

h. between muscles

i. bursitis

j. dorsiflexion

k. rheumatoid arthritis

l. rotation

m. eversion

n. rheumatic fever

o. subtendinous bursae

C. Key Terms

Use the text to look up the following terms. Write the definition or explanation.

49. Abduction:

_____

_____

50. Adduction:

_____

_____

51. Amphiarthrosis:

_____

_____

52. Articulation:

_____

_____

53. Ball-and-socket joint:

_____

_____

54. Bursae:

_____

_____

55. Circumduction:

_____

_____

56. Condyloid joint:

_____

_____

57. Depression:

_____

_____

58. Diarthroses or synovial joints:

_____

_____

59. Dorsiflexion:

_____

_____

60. Elevation:

_____

_____

61. Eversion:

_____

_____

62. Extension:

_____

_____

63. Fascia:

_____

_____

64. Flexion:

_____

_____

65. Gliding joint:

_____

_____

66. Gomphosis:

_____

_____

67. Hinge joint:

_____

_____

68. Hyperextension:

_____

_____

69. Inversion:

_____

_____

70. Opposition:

_____

_____

71. Osteoarthritis:

_____

_____

72. Pivot joint:

_____

_____

73. Plantar flexion:

_____

_____

74. Primary fibrositis:

_____

_____

75. Pronation:

_____

_____

76. Protraction:

_____

_____

77. Reposition:

_____

_____

78. Retraction:

_____

_____

79. Rotation:

_____

_____

80. Saddle joint:

_____

_____

81. Subcutaneous bursae:

_____

_____

82. Subfascial bursae:

_____

_____

83. Subtendinous bursae:

_____

_____

84. Supination:

_____

_____

85. Suture:

_____

_____

86. Symphysis:

_____

_____

87. Synarthroses:

_____

_____

88. Synchondrosis:

_____

_____

89. Syndesmosis:

_____

_____

D. Labeling Exercise

90. Label the joints as indicated in Figure 8-1.

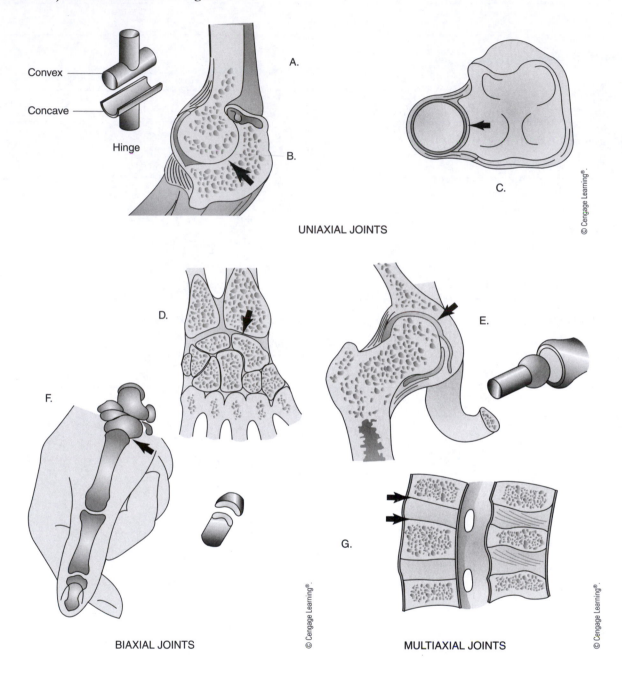

Figure 8-1

A. _____   E. _____

B. _____   F. _____

C. _____   G. _____

D. _____

91. Label the parts of the knee joint as indicated in Figure 8-2.

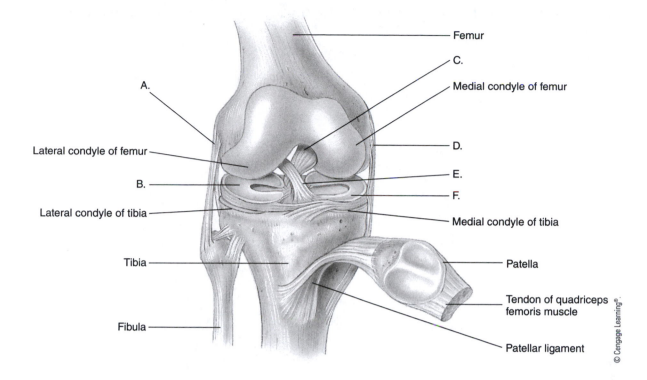

Figure 8-2

A. _____

B. _____

C. _____

D. _____

E. _____

F. _____

E. Coloring Exercise

92. Using Figure 8-3, color the bones red, the articular cartilage blue, the synovial membrane green, and the synovial fluid yellow.

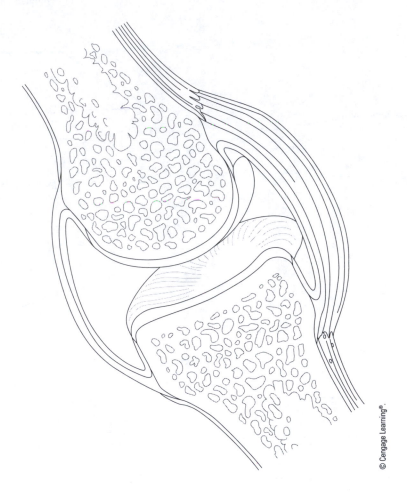

© Cengage Learning®.

Figure 8-3

F. Critical Thinking

Answer the following questions in complete sentences.

93. What are the criteria for classifying joints?

94. Why do some authors consider syndesmosis an example of amphiarthrosis?

95. Differentiate amphiarthrosis and diarthrosis.

96. Why does the shoulder joint have the greatest range of motion?

97. Why is moderate, regular exercise important as we age?

98. Why are primates the only animals to use hand tools?

99. What is meant by uniaxial, biaxial, and multiaxial?

100. Of the three types of bursae, which would be least likely to have bursitis? Explain.

101. Why would rheumatic fever affect the heart?

G. Crossword Puzzle

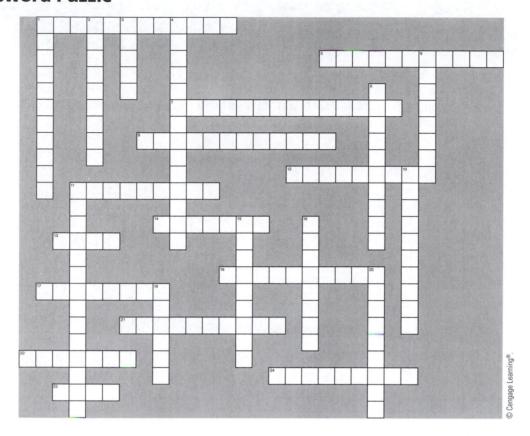

Complete the crossword puzzle using the following clues.

ACROSS

1. Immovable joint
5. Synovial joints
7. Joints with slight movement
9. Joint
11. Palm down
12. Sole in
13. Hinge joint
14. Condyloid joint
17. Inflamed bursa
19. Ball-and-socket joint
21. Move a part backward
22. Decreasing the angle between joints
23. Excessive uric acid
24. Buffer between vertebrae

DOWN

1. Bones move as one
2. Inflamed joint
3. Saddle joint
4. Degenerative joint disease
6. Around an axis
8. Lower a part
10. Motion unique to the thumb
11. Foot pushes down
15. Toward the midline
16. Bone-to-bone connector
18. Joints of skull
20. Synovial fluid

CASE STUDY

Denzel, a 46-year-old man, is working with his physical therapist on a set of back exercises. Around 4 weeks ago, Denzel was helping a friend move and attempted to lift a heavy box. Since that incident, he has had severe pain in his lower back. His health care provider prescribed physical therapy three times per week to treat the condition.

QUESTIONS

1. What condition might Denzel be suffering from?

2. What can cause this condition to develop?

3. What treatment might be considered if Denzel does not respond to physical therapy?

CHAPTER QUIZ

1. Joints are classified into how many major groups?

   a. 1   d. 4
   b. 2   e. 5
   c. 3

Answer:

2. In a suture, the bones are united by

   a. ligaments   d. adipose tissue
   b. tendons   e. fibrous tissue
   c. epithelial tissue

Answer:

3. In a syndesmosis joint, the bursae are united by

   a. ligaments   d. adipose tissue
   b. tendons   e. fibrous tissue
   c. epithelial tissue

Answer:

4. A tooth is an example of a(n)

   a. synchondrosis   d. gomphosis
   b. diarthrosis   e. symphysis
   c. amphiarthrosis

Answer:

5. A joint in which the bones are connected by a disk of fibrocartilage is a

   a. synchondrosis
   b. diarthrosis
   c. synarthrosis

   d. gomphosis
   e. symphysis

Answer:

6. Two bony surfaces are connected by hyaline cartilage; this is a

   a. synchondrosis
   b. diarthrosis
   c. synarthrosis

   d. gomphosis
   e. symphysis

Answer:

7. Cartilage supplying a smooth, gliding surface is

   a. fibrous
   b. aponeurosis
   c. articular

   d. hyaline
   e. collagenous

Answer:

8. Material connecting one bone to another and forming a joint capsule is

   a. ligamentous
   b. collagenous
   c. tendinous

   d. adipose
   e. cartilaginous

Answer:

9. The femur joins with the tibia at its distal end and fits into what at its proximal end?

   a. glenoid fossa
   b. symphysis
   c. carpal

   d. acetabulum
   e. none of the above

Answer:

10. The proximal end of the femur is attached at the joint by

    a. tendons
    b. ligaments
    c. cartilage

    d. collagen
    e. none of the above

Answer:

11. Which of the following movements is possible in a synarthrosis joint?

    a. flexion
    b. rotation
    c. abduction

    d. opposition
    e. none of the above

Answer:

12. With circumduction, the bone movement is a circle and a(n)

    a. square
    b. extension
    c. cone

    d. rotation
    e. none of the above

Answer:

13. The opposite of abduction is

    a. circumduction
    b. adduction
    c. flexion

    d. dorsiflexion
    e. none of the above

Answer:

14. The opposite of dorsiflexion is

    a. extension
    b. adduction
    c. inversion

    d. plantar flexion
    e. none of the above

Answer:

15. Supination and pronation refer to movement of the

    a. foot and ankle
    b. knee and hip
    c. wrist and elbow

    d. shoulder and spine
    e. none of the above

Answer:

16. If the palm is moved from posterior to anterior, this is an example of

    a. inversion
    b. supination
    c. pronation

    d. rotation
    e. none of the above

Answer:

17. Opposition is unique to

    a. primates
    b. man
    c. mammals

    d. apes
    e. none of the above

Answer:

18. The number of diarthroses or synovial joints is

    a. 2
    b. 4
    c. 6

    d. 8
    e. none of the above

Answer:

19. A convex surface fits into a concave surface. What kind of joint is this?

    a. hinge
    b. condyloid
    c. pivot

    d. saddle
    e. gliding

Answer:

20. An ellipsoidal joint is also known as which type of joint?

    a. hinge
    b. condyloid
    c. pivot

    d. saddle
    e. gliding

Answer:

21. The type of joint formed by opposing planes surfaces is a

    a. hinge
    b. condyloid
    c. pivot
    d. saddle
    e. gliding

Answer:

22. The joint allowing for thumb opposition is the

    a. hinge
    b. condyloid
    c. pivot
    d. saddle
    e. gliding

Answer:

23. Subfascial bursae are located between

    a. bones
    b. muscles
    c. ligaments
    d. tendon
    e. skin and bone

Answer:

24. Subcutaneous bursae are found between

    a. bones
    b. muscles
    c. ligaments
    d. tendons
    e. skin and bone

Answer:

25. Subtendinous bursae are found between

    a. bones
    b. muscles
    c. ligaments
    d. tendons
    e. skin and bone

Answer:

26. Synovial sac inflammation is

    a. bursitis
    b. arthritis
    c. osteoarthritis
    d. gout
    e. primary fibrositis

Answer:

27. Total joint inflammation is

    a. bursitis
    b. arthritis
    c. osteoarthritis
    d. gout
    e. primary fibrositis

Answer:

28. Lumbago is

    a. bursitis
    b. arthritis
    c. osteoarthritis
    d. gout
    e. primary fibrositis

Answer:

29. Which of the following causes joint degeneration?

    a. bursitis
    b. arthritis
    c. osteoarthritis

    d. gout
    e. primary fibrositis

Answer:

30. Which of the following can cause kidney damage?

    a. bursitis
    b. arthritis
    c. osteoarthritis

    d. gout
    e. primary fibrositis

Answer:

31. A slipped disk is also referred to as (a)

    a. herniated disk
    b. arthritis
    c. gout

    d. sprain
    e. primary fibrositis

Answer:

32. The joint between the atlas vertebra and the axis vertebra is an example of which type of joint?

    a. pivot
    b. saddle
    c. ball and socket

    d. gliding
    e. hinge

Answer:

33. Synovial fluid has two functions: creating a gliding surface and nourishing

    a. articular cartilage
    b. fascia
    c. muscles

    d. white blood cells
    e. spongy bone

Answer:

The Muscular System

OBJECTIVES

After studying this chapter, you should be able to:

1. Describe the gross and microscopic anatomy of skeletal muscle.

2. Describe and compare the basic differences between the anatomy of skeletal, smooth, and cardiac muscle.

3. Explain the current concept of muscle contraction based on three factors: neuroelectrical, chemical, and energy sources.

4. Define *muscle tone* and compare isotonic and isometric contractions.

5. List factors that can cause muscles to malfunction, causing various disorders.

6. Name and identify the location of major superficial muscles of the body.

ACTIVITIES

A. Completion

Fill in the blank spaces with the correct term.

1. Skeletal muscle is striated and ___.

2. Because their length is greater than their width, skeletal muscle cells are referred to as muscle ___.

3. The sarcolemma is surrounded by three types of connective tissue; they are the ___, the ___, and the ___.

4. A bands are the ___ bands, and I bands are the ___ bands.

5. There are no cross-bridges in the ___.

6. The actual process of contraction occurs in the area called the ___.

7. Muscle fibrils are surrounded by membranes in the form of ___ and ___.

NAME: _____   DATE: _____

8. These structures are referred to as the ___ system.

9. An irregular curtain around each of the fibrils is the ___ ___.

10. A motor unit is innervated by a(n) ___ ___.

11. Each motor unit in the ___ muscle contains about 10 muscle cells.

12. A muscle fiber's membrane is surrounded by ___.

13. The two minerals causing a resting potential in a muscle are ___ and ___.

14. The electrical potential is caused by a rapid influx of ___ ions.

15. A muscle cell generating its own impulse is called its ___ ___.

16. The two inhibitor substances surrounding the actin are ___ and ___.

17. The substance negating their effect is ___.

18. The discoverer of the protein myosin was ___.

19. During contraction, the width of the A bands remains constant while the ___ move closer.

20. The four sources of ATP for the energy of contraction are ___, ___, ___ ___ ___, and ___ plus two ATP.

21. The all-or-none law states that a muscle contraction either ___ or it ___ ___.

22. A constant state of partial contraction is called ___.

23. The muscle that is nonstriated and found in hollow structures is ___.

24. Smooth muscle contraction occurs without the regular rearrangement of ___.

25. Cardiac muscle is under the control of the ___ nervous system.

26. Fibrillation of cardiac muscle can result in ___.

27. Prime movers are ___.

28. ___ assist the prime movers.

29. Muscles found directly under the skin are ___ muscles.

30. ___ is muscle pain.

31. Doctors of ___ medicine take a therapeutic approach to medicine by placing greater emphasis on the relationship between the organs and the musculoskeletal system.

32. ___ is a form of rheumatism but does not affect the joints.

33. Stepping on an old nail can transfer the bacterium causing ___ to body tissues.

B. Matching

Match the term on the right with the definition on the left.

_____ 34. striated muscle

_____ 35. electrical cell membrane

_____ 36. delicate connective tissue

_____ 37. individual bundles of cells

_____ 38. surrounds whole muscle

_____ 39. dark bands of protein

_____ 40. light of protein

_____ 41. forms irregular curtain

_____ 42. inside minus outside plus

a. resting potential

b. phosphocreatine

c. trapezius

d. myosin

e. isotonic contraction

f. origin

g. fibrillation

h. insertion

i. skeletal

_____ 43. muscle impulse

_____ 44. contain ATP molecule

_____ 45. only in muscle tissue

_____ 46. tension remains the same

_____ 47. rapid uncontrolled contraction

_____ 48. fixed attachment of muscle

_____ 49. movable attachment of muscle

_____ 50. prime mover

_____ 51. draw scalp backward

_____ 52. smiling muscle

_____ 53. between the neck and clavicle

j. fascicle

k. action potential

l. sarcolemma

m. actin

n. zygomaticus

o. sarcoplasmic reticulum

p. myosin filaments

q. endomysium

r. epimysium

s. agonists

t. occipitalis

C. Key Terms

Use the text to look up the following terms. Write the definition or explanation.

54. A bands:

_____

_____

55. Abductor digiti minimi:

_____

_____

56. Abductor hallucis:

_____

_____

57. Abductor pollicis:

_____

_____

58. Acetylcholine:

_____

_____

59. Actin:

_____

_____

60. Action potential:

_____

_____

61. Adductor pollicis:

_____

_____

62. Agonists:

_____

_____

63. All-or-none law:

_____

_____

64. Anconeus:

_____

_____

65. Antagonists:

_____

_____

66. Aponeurosis:

_____

_____

67. Biceps femoris:

_____

_____

68. Brachialis:

_____

_____

69. Buccinator:

_____

_____

70. Cardiac muscle:

_____

_____

71. Contracture:

_____

_____

72. Cramps:

_____

_____

73. Deltoid:

_____

_____

74. Diaphragm:

_____

_____

75. Electrical potential:

_____

_____

76. Endomysium:

_____

_____

77. Epimysium:

_____

_____

78. Extensor carpi:

_____

_____

79. Extensor digitorum:

_____

_____

80. Extensor hallucis:

_____

_____

81. Extensor pollicis:

_____

_____

82. External intercostals:

_____

_____

83. External oblique:

_____

_____

84. Fascia:

_____

_____

85. Fascicle:

_____

_____

86. Fasciculi:

_____

_____

87. Fibrillation:

_____

_____

88. Flexor carpi:

_____

_____

89. Flexor digitorum:

_____

_____

90. Flexor hallucis:

_____

_____

91. Flexor pollicis:

_____

_____

92. Frontalis:

_____

_____

93. Gastrocnemius:

_____

_____

94. Gluteus maximus:

_____

_____

95. Gluteus medius:

_____

_____

96. Gluteus minimus:

_____

_____

97. Gracilis:

_____

_____

98. H band:

_____

_____

99. Hypertrophy:

_____

_____

100. I band:

_____

_____

101. Iliacus:

_____

_____

102. Inferior oblique:

_____

_____

103. Inferior rectus:

_____

_____

104. Infraspinatus:

_____

_____

105. Insertion:

_____

_____

106. Internal intercostals:

_____

_____

107. Internal oblique:

_____

_____

108. Interossei:

_____

_____

109. Isometric activity:

_____

_____

110. Isotonic activity:

_____

_____

111. Lateral rectus:

_____

_____

112. Latissimus dorsi:

_____

_____

113. Levator labii superioris:

_____

_____

114. Levator scapulae:

_____

_____

115. Masseter:

_____

_____

116. Mastication:

_____

_____

117. Medial rectus:

_____

_____

118. Motor unit:

_____

_____

119. Muscle twitch:

_____

_____

120. Myalgia:

_____

_____

121. Myosin:

_____

_____

122. Occipitalis:

_____

_____

123. Opponens pollicis:

_____

_____

124. Orbicularis oris:

_____

_____

125. Origin:

_____

_____

126. Pectoralis major:

_____

_____

127. Pectoralis minor:

_____

_____

128. Perimysium:

_____

_____

129. Peroneus longus:

_____

_____

130. Peroneus tertius:

_____

_____

131. Phosphocreatine:

_____

_____

132. Plantar fasciitis:

_____

_____

133. Plantaris:

_____

_____

134. Polio:

_____

_____

135. Popliteus:

_____

_____

136. Pronator quadratus:

_____

_____

137. Pronator teres:

_____

_____

138. Psoas:

_____

_____

139. Pterygoid:

_____

_____

140. Quadriceps femoris:

_____

_____

141. Rectus abdominis:

_____

_____

142. Rectus femoris:

_____

_____

143. Resting potential:

_____

_____

144. Rhomboids:

_____

_____

145. Rigor mortis:

_____

_____

146. Sarcolemma:

_____

_____

147. Sarcomere:

_____

_____

148. Sarcoplasmic reticulum:

_____

_____

149. Sarcotubular system:

_____

_____

150. Sartorius:

_____

_____

151. Semimembranosus:

_____

_____

152. Semitendinosus:

_____

_____

153. Serratus anterior:

_____

_____

154. Skeletal muscle:

_____

_____

155. Smooth muscle:

_____

_____

156. Soleus:

_____

_____

157. Sternocleidomastoid:

_____

_____

158. Superior oblique:

_____

_____

159. Superior rectus:

_____

_____

160. Supinator:

_____

_____

161. Supraspinatus:

_____

_____

162. Synergists:

_____

_____

163. Sartorius:

_____

_____

164. Semimembranosus:

_____

_____

165. Semitendinosus:

_____

_____

166. Serratus anterior:

_____

_____

167. Skeletal muscle:

_____

_____

168. Smooth muscle:

_____

_____

169. Soleus:

_____

_____

170. Sternocleidomastoid:

_____

_____

171. Superior oblique:

_____

_____

172. Superior rectus:

_____

_____

173. Supinator:

_____

_____

174. Supraspinatus:

_____

_____

175. T system:

_____

_____

176. Vastus intermedius:

_____

_____

177. Vastus lateralis:

_____

_____

178. Vastus medialis:

_____

_____

179. Z line:

_____

_____

180. Zygomaticus:

_____

_____

D. Labeling Exercise

181. Label the superficial muscles as indicated in Figure 9-1.

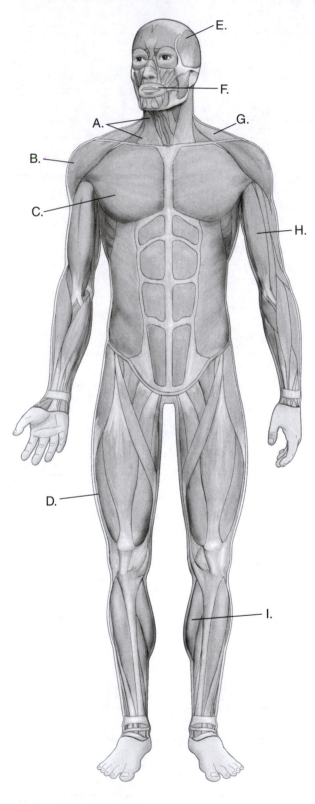

A. _____

B. _____

C. _____

D. _____

E. _____

F. _____

G. _____

H. _____

I. _____

Figure 9-1

182. Label the superficial muscles as indicated in Figure 9-2.

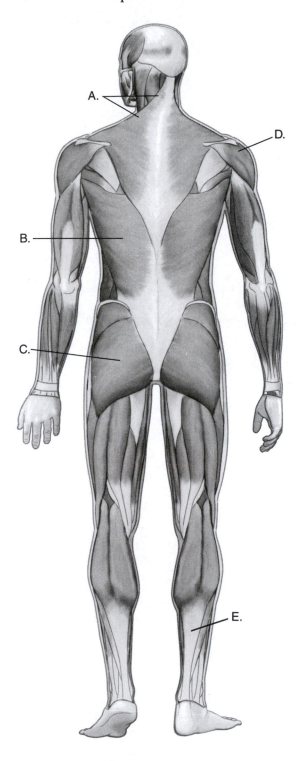

A. _____

B. _____

C. _____

D. _____

E. _____

Figure 9-2

E. Coloring Exercise

183. Using Figure 9-3, color the gluteus maximus red, the biceps femoris (long head) blue, the biceps femoris (short head) yellow, the soleus green, and the calcaneal tendon orange.

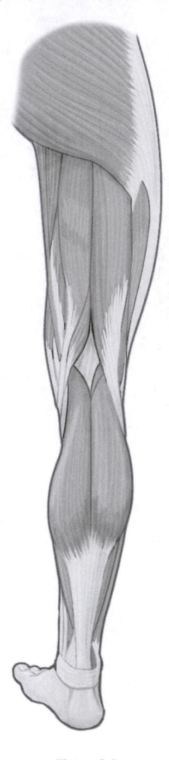

Figure 9-3

F. Critical Thinking

Answer the following questions in complete sentences.

184. Why should weightlifters do aerobic exercises for maximal physical fitness?

185. Explain two ways in which prolonged exertion during hot weather might cause muscles to malfunction.

186. Why does stimulation of nerves with electrical current help stave off muscle atrophy for a short period of time?

187. Explain the function of troponin and tropomyosin and what negates them.

188. On what does the strength of contractions depend? Explain.

189. Identify age-related changes in the muscle system. Explain what a sports medicine physician and a massage therapist can do to help.

G. Crossword Puzzle

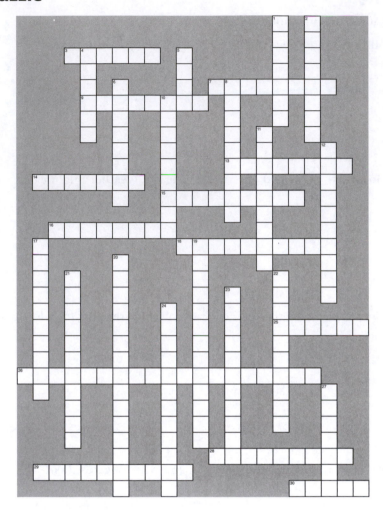

Complete the crossword puzzle using the following clues.

ACROSS

3. Muscle found in hollow body structures
7. Contraction when lifting a weight
9. Skeletal muscle type
13. Muscle that closes the jaw
14. Muscle pain
15. Movable muscle attachment
16. Muscle that protrudes the lower lip
18. Electrically polarized cell membrane
25. Fixed muscle attachment
26. Muscle that moves the head
28. Activity from tension against muscles

DOWN

1. Injection site in the arm
2. Muscle inflammation
4. Thick protein filament in muscle cells
5. Constant state of partial contraction
6. Inhibitor substance
8. Area between Z lines
10. Muscle between the neck and clavicle
11. Skeletal muscle bundles
12. Muscle that raises the mandible
17. Muscles that assist the prime mover
19. Neurotransmitter substance

29. Muscle that compresses the cheek

30. Thin filaments of protein

20. Rapid source of high-energy ATP

21. Increase in muscle size

22. Actin united with myosin

23. Smiling and laughing muscles

24. Rapid, uncontrolled contraction of heart cells

27. Prime mover

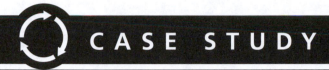

CASE STUDY

Nadea, a 35-year-old woman, tells the nurse practitioner at the local clinic that she is having problems holding her eyes open, smiling, and keeping her lips closed. She also states that she feels generally weak and easily fatigued. The nurse notes that Nadea has droopy eyelids and her face has little expression.

QUESTIONS

1. What condition might be causing Nadea's symptoms of muscle fatigue and weakness?

2. What muscles does this disorder affect first?

3. Why does this condition develop?

CHAPTER QUIZ

1. Muscles make up what percentage of body weight?

   a. 10–20%
   b. 20–30%
   c. 30–40%
   d. 40–50%
   e. 50–60%

Answer:

2. The longest and most slender muscle fibers are

   a. smooth
   b. skeletal
   c. cardiac
   d. uninucleated
   e. none of the above

Answer:

3. The entire muscle consists of a number of skeletal muscle bundles called

   a. perimysium
   b. myosin
   c. fasciculi

   d. actin
   e. none of the above

Answer:

4. The sarcomere is the area between two

   a. Z bands
   b. H bands
   c. I bands

   d. A bands
   e. none of the above

Answer:

5. The layer of areolar tissue covering the whole muscle trunk is called

   a. fascicle
   b. fasciculi
   c. epimysium

   d. fascia
   e. none of the above

Answer:

6. The light bands are the

   a. A bands
   b. Z lines
   c. H bands

   d. I bands
   e. none of the above

Answer:

7. The sarcotubular system is made up of the sarcoplasmic reticulum and the

   a. T system
   b. H system
   c. sarcomere

   d. vesicle system
   e. none of the above

Answer:

8. On the average, a single motor nerve fiber innervates about how many muscle cells?

   a. 100
   b. 150
   c. 200

   d. 250
   e. none of the above

Answer:

9. Which of the following properties do muscle cells NOT possess?

   a. excitability
   b. conductivity
   c. contractility

   d. elasticity
   e. none of the above

Answer:

10. Which of the following is a neurotransmitter?

    a. acetylcholine
    b. myosin
    c. actin

    d. tropomyosin
    e. none of the above

Answer:

11. Muscle contraction is

    a. resting potential
    b. electrical potential
    c. action potential

    d. chemical potential
    e. none of the above

Answer:

12. Calcium negates the effect of

    a. myosin
    b. troponin
    c. actin

    d. sodium
    e. none of the above

Answer:

13. The sodium–potassium pump restores

    a. resting potential
    b. electrical potential
    c. action potential

    d. chemical potential
    e. none of the above

Answer:

14. Actin was discovered in

    a. 1868
    b. 1934
    c. 1942

    d. 1960
    e. none of the above

Answer:

15. Which of the following retains the same width during contraction?

    a. A bands
    b. I bands
    c. H bands

    d. Z lines
    e. none of the above

Answer:

16. Which of the following moves apart at the end of a contraction?

    a. A bands
    b. I bands
    c. H bands

    d. Z lines
    e. none of the above

Answer:

17. ATP is synthesized by all of the following EXCEPT

    a. glycolysis
    b. Krebs citric acid cycle
    c. electron transport

    d. breakdown of phosphocreatine
    e. none of the above

Answer:

18. Which of the following is a rapid source of high-energy ATP for muscle contraction?

    a. glycolysis
    b. Krebs citric acid cycle
    c. electron transport

    d. breakdown of phosphocreatine
    e. none of the above

Answer:

19. Which of the following does a contraction NOT depend on?

    a. strength of stimulus
    b. duration of stimulus
    c. speed of stimulus
    d. temperature
    e. none of the above

Answer:

20. Muscle remains at constant length but tension increases. What type of contraction is this?

    a. isotonic
    b. isometric
    c. tonal
    d. internal
    e. none of the above

Answer:

21. Muscle shortens and thickens while tension remains constant. What type of contraction is this?

    a. isotonic
    b. isometric
    c. tonal
    d. internal
    e. none of the above

Answer:

22. Some muscles will always be contracting while others are at rest. What type of contraction is this?

    a. isotonic
    b. isometric
    c. tonal
    d. external
    e. none of the above

Answer:

23. Two of the three kinds of muscle in the body are uninucleated; they are

    a. smooth and cardiac
    b. smooth and skeletal
    c. cardiac and skeletal
    d. visceral and striated
    e. none of the above

Answer:

24. Contraction is fastest in which kind of muscle?

    a. smooth
    b. cardiac
    c. skeletal
    d. visceral
    e. none of the above

Answer:

25. The wide, flat attachment of muscle to bone is called

    a. ligament
    b. tendon
    c. insertion
    d. aponeurosis
    e. origin

Answer:

26. The attachment of the biceps to the forearm is the

    a. agonist
    b. insertion
    c. origin
    d. ligament
    e. none of above

Answer:

27. Muscles that straighten a joint are called

    a. agonists
    b. synergists
    c. insertions
    d. antagonists
    e. origins

Answer:

28. An increase in muscle size is called

    a. atrophy
    b. myositis
    c. hypertrophy
    d. myalgia
    e. myasthenia gravis

Answer:

29. Muscle weakness is called

    a. atrophy
    b. myositis
    c. hypertrophy
    d. myalgia
    e. myasthenia gravis

Answer:

30. Inflammation of muscle tissue is called

    a. atrophy
    b. myositis
    c. hypertrophy
    d. myalgia
    e. myasthenia gravis

Answer:

31. In the 1940s and 1950s, many children developed paralysis of their limbs and had to be placed in "iron lungs" after contracting

    a. myalgia
    b. plantar fasciitis
    c. tetanus
    d. myositis
    e. polio

Answer:

32. Which of the following muscles extends the thigh?

    a. adductor magnus
    b. abductor brevis
    c. tensor fascia lata
    d. adductor longus
    e. sartorius

Answer:

33. The main muscles that close the jaw are the temporalis and the

    a. superior rectus
    b. masseter
    c. pterygoid
    d. buccinator
    e. orbicularis oris

Answer:

CHAPTER 10

The Nervous System: Introduction, Spinal Cord, and Spinal Nerves

OBJECTIVES

After studying this chapter, you should be able to:

1. Name the major subdivisions of the nervous system.
2. Classify the different types of neuroglia cells.
3. List the structural and functional classification of neurons.
4. Explain how a neuron transmits a nerve impulse.
5. Name the different types of neural tissues and their definitions.
6. Describe the structure of the spinal cord.
7. Name and number the spinal nerves.

ACTIVITIES

A. Completion

Fill in the blank spaces with the correct term.

1. Being a(n) ___ center and a(n) ___ network is a function of the nervous system.
2. The control center for the entire system is the ___ ___ ___.
3. The sensory system, also named the ___ ___ ___, is a subdivision of the ___ ___ ___.
4. Motor neurons are part of the ___ ___ ___.
5. The speeding up of activity is a function of the ___ portion of the ANS.

NAME: _____   DATE: _____

6. ___ slows down the system, whereas ___ speeds it up.

7. A nerve is a bundle of ___.

8. The nerve glue is the ___ cell.

9. ___ cells form myelin sheaths around nerve fibers.

10. The star-shaped ___ prevents toxic substances from entering the brain.

11. Protein synthesis occurs in the ___ ___, also called ___ ___.

12. The branches of trees on the nerve cell are the ___.

13. Peripheral axons are enclosed in fatty ___ sheaths.

14. Most neurons of the brain are ___.

15. Myelin gaps are called ___.

16. The transmission of impulses is handled by the ___ neurons.

17. The efferent neurons are multipolar; the afferent neurons are ___.

18. The act of salivating would be caused by a(n) ___ neuron.

19. The three types of ions involved in nerve impulses are ___, ___, and ___.

20. Reversal of electrical charge is ___.

21. When the outside of a nerve is positively charged and the inside is negatively charged, the condition is known as the ___ ___.

22. The nerve impulse is a self-propagating wave of ___.

23. The gap between the axon of one nerve and the dendrite of another is referred to as the ___.

24. The impulse is carried across the gap by ___.

25. An involuntary reaction to an external stimulus is called a(n) ___.

26. The gray matter on the brain's surface is known as the ___.

27. The spider layer of the meninges is the ___ ___.

28. The sensory root of the spinal cord is the ___ ___.

29. There are ___ pairs of cervical nerves.

30. External stimuli affect ___ neurons.

31. One example of a(n) ___ is Valium.

32. Taken in large doses, anabolic steroids have a(n) ___ feedback effect on the hypothalamus.

33. The transparent fibrous membrane that forms a tube around the spinal cord is the ___ ___.

B. Matching

Match the term on the right with the definition on the left.

_____ 34. control center

_____ 35. motor neuron

_____ 36. sensory neurons

_____ 37. majority of brain cells

_____ 38. neurons with multiple dendrites

a. reflex

b. adrenaline

c. pia mater

d. neurofibril nodes

e. synapse

_____ 39. neurolemmocytes

_____ 40. myelin sheath gaps

_____ 41. association neuron

_____ 42. creates action potential

_____ 43. gap between neurons

_____ 44. epinephrine

_____ 45. involuntary reaction

_____ 46. like male hormones

_____ 47. fiber bundle inside the CNS

_____ 48. delicate mother

_____ 49. spinal gray matter

_____ 50. dorsal root

_____ 51. ventral root

_____ 52. C1–C8

_____ 53. phagocytosis of microbes

f. cervical nerves

g. horn

h. anabolic steroids

i. CNS

j. efferent

k. internuncial

l. sensory

m. microglia

n. depolarization

o. neuroglia

p. tract

q. afferent

r. motor

s. Schwann cells

t. multipolar

C. Key Terms

Use the text to look up the following terms. Write the definition or explanation.

54. Acetylcholine:

_____

_____

55. Acetylcholinesterase:

_____

_____

56. Action potential:

_____

_____

57. Adrenaline/epinephrine:

_____

_____

58. Afferent peripheral system:

_____

_____

59. All-or-none law:

_____

_____

60. Anterior or ventral gray horn:

_____

_____

61. Arachnoid mater:

_____

_____

62. Astrocytes:

_____

_____

63. Autonomic nervous system:

_____

_____

64. Axon:

_____

_____

65. Axon terminals:

_____

_____

66. Bipolar neurons:

_____

_____

67. Central nervous system (CNS):

_____

_____

68. Chromatophilic substance or Nissl bodies:

_____

_____

69. Cortex:

_____

_____

70. Dendrites:

_____

_____

71. Depolarization:

_____

_____

72. Dopamine:

_____

_____

73. Dura mater:

_____

_____

74. Efferent peripheral system:

_____

_____

75. Endorphins:

_____

_____

76. Ependymal cells:

_____

_____

77. Ganglia:

_____

_____

78. Glial cells:

_____

_____

79. Gray matter:

_____

_____

80. Horns:

_____

_____

81. Internuncial or association neurons:

_____

_____

82. Membrane or resting potential:

_____

_____

83. Meninges:

_____

_____

84. Microglial cells:

_____

_____

85. Motor or efferent neuron:

_____

_____

86. Multipolar neurons:

_____

_____

87. Myelin sheath:

_____

_____

88. Nerve:

_____

_____

89. Neuroglia:

_____

_____

90. Neurons:

_____

_____

91. Nodes of Ranvier/neurofibril nodes:

_____

_____

92. Norepinephrine:

_____

_____

93. Nucleus:

_____

_____

94. Oligodendroglia:

_____

_____

95. Parasympathetic division:

_____

_____

96. Peripheral nervous system (PNS):

_____

_____

97. Pia mater:

_____

_____

98. Posterior or dorsal gray horn:

_____

_____

99. Posterior or dorsal root:

_____

_____

100. Reflex:

_____

_____

101. Reflex arc:

_____

_____

102. Repolarization:

_____

_____

103. Schwann cells/neurolemmocytes:

_____

_____

104. Sensory or afferent neuron:

_____

_____

105. Serotonin:

_____

_____

106. Somatic nervous system:

_____

_____

107. Spinal meninges:

_____

_____

108. Sympathetic division:

_____

_____

109. Synapses:

_____

_____

110. Tract:

_____

_____

111. Unipolar neurons:

_____

_____

112. Ventral root:

_____

_____

113. White matter:

_____

_____

D. Labeling Exercise

114. Label the nerve cells as indicated in Figure 10-1.

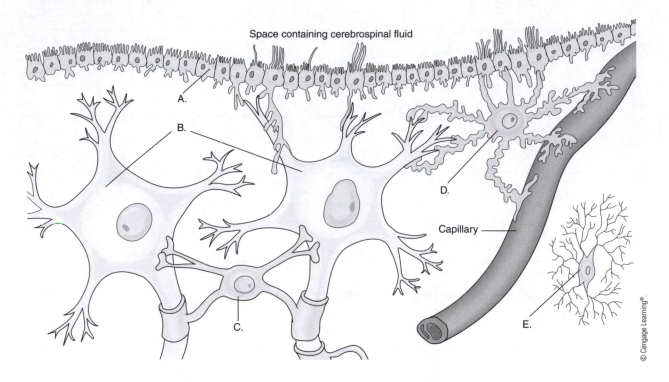

Figure 10-1

A. _____

B. _____

C. _____

D. _____

E. _____

115. Label the parts of the neuron as indicated in Figure 10-2.

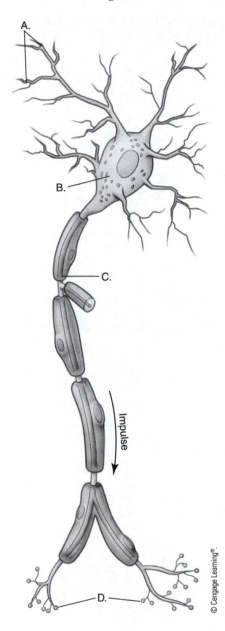

Figure 10-2

A. _____

B. _____

C. _____

D. _____

E. _____

E. Coloring Exercise

116. Using Figure 10-3, color the cervical spinal nerves red, the thoracic spinal nerves green, the lumbar spinal nerves yellow, and the sacral spinal nerves blue.

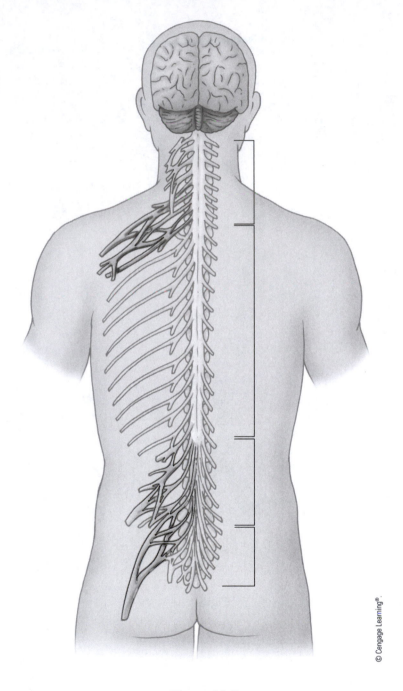

Figure 10-3

© Cengage Learning®.

F. Critical Thinking

Answer the following questions in complete sentences.

117. Explain how the sympathetic and parasympathetic systems work during a "fight-or-flight" experience.

118. Why is an efferent neuron multipolar?

119. Why do myelin-covered neurons carry an action potential faster than an uncovered neuron?

120. Why doesn't acetylcholine remain on the postsynaptic neuron?

121. Using the five components of the reflex arc, explain the body's reaction to a hand on a hot surface.

122. How does the reflex action help maintain homeostasis?

G. Crossword Puzzle

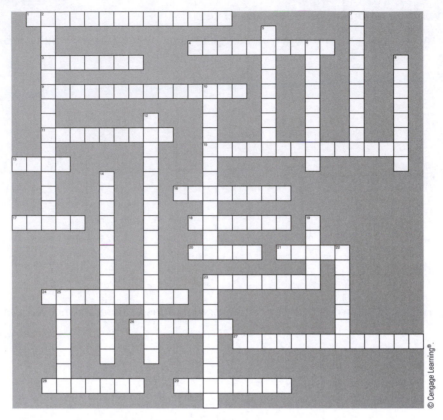

Complete the crossword puzzle using the following clues.

ACROSS

1. Sympathetic neurotransmitter
3. Nerve cell groups
4. Neurons that have several dendrites and one axon
9. Creates action potential
11. Receive stimuli
13. Long extension of a nerve cell body
15. Recharge nerves
16. Protective membrane
17. Bundle inside the CNS
18. One axon, one dendrite
20. Cells that support and protect
21. Gray matter in spinal cord
23. Resting potential
24. Star shaped
26. Afferent neuron
27. Uppers
28. Nerve cells
29. Cells with only one process

DOWN

2. Semirigid rows
5. Line brain ventricles
6. Spider layer
7. Downer
8. Motor neuron
10. Association neuron
12. Serotonin, endorphins
14. Parasympathetic neurotransmitter
19. Bundle of nerve cells
22. Kind of cells that form myelin sheaths
23. Do phagocytosis
25. Gap between neurons

CASE STUDY

Lalia Escobar, a 20-year-old pre-medical student, is scheduled to undergo a spinal tap this morning for diagnostic purposes. Lalia has been instructed about the procedure by her health care providers. Lalia learns that cerebrospinal fluid will be extracted during the spinal tap and sent to the laboratory for analysis.

QUESTIONS

1. When performing a spinal tap, where must the needle be inserted in order to avoid damage to the spinal cord?

2. What can health care providers learn from analysis of a patient's cerebrospinal fluid?

3. In addition to analyzing cerebrospinal fluid, what are other purposes for a spinal tap?

CHAPTER QUIZ

1. The nervous system shares in the maintenance of homeostasis with which system?

a. respiratory
b. endocrine
c. skeletal
d. digestive
e. muscular

Answer:

2. The system that conducts impulses from the brain and spinal cord to skeletal muscles is the

a. parasympathetic
b. sympathetic
c. autonomic
d. somatic
e. afferent

Answer:

3. The "glue" cells that perform the function of support and protection are

a. neurons
b. astrocytes
c. neuroglia
d. ependymal
e. Schwann

Answer:

4. Oligodendroglia are found in the

a. brain and spinal cord
b. heart
c. fingers
d. muscles
e. lungs

Answer:

5. Phagocytosis is performed by

   a. astrocytes
   b. oligodendroglia
   c. microglia

   d. ependymal cells
   e. Schwann cells

Answer:

6. The cells that make up the myelin sheath are

   a. astrocytes
   b. oligodendroglia
   c. microglia

   d. ependymal cells
   e. Schwann cells

Answer:

7. The cells that line the cavities in brain and spinal cord are

   a. astrocytes
   b. oligodendroglia
   c. microglia

   d. ependymal cells
   e. Schwann cells

Answer:

8. Nissl bodies are attached to

   a. mitochondria
   b. endoplasmic reticulum
   c. lysosome

   d. Golgi bodies
   e. neurofibrils

Answer:

9. Neurolemmocytes are also known as

   a. astrocytes
   b. oligodendroglia
   c. microglia

   d. ependymal cells
   e. Schwann cells

Answer:

10. A neuron with one axon and one dendrite is known as

    a. unipolar
    b. bipolar
    c. afferent

    d. multipolar
    e. terminal

Answer:

11. Receptors are

    a. afferent neurons
    b. efferent neurons
    c. multipolar neurons

    d. association neurons
    e. internuncial neurons

Answer:

12. Reaction neurons are

    a. afferent neurons
    b. efferent neurons
    c. association neurons

    d. unipolar neurons
    e. internuncial neurons

Answer:

13. The sodium pump is used to maintain the

    a. action potential
    b. electrical potential
    c. membrane

    d. depolarization
    e. repolarization

Answer:

14. Which of the following is NOT a neurotransmitter?

    a. acetylcholine
    b. norepinephrine
    c. serotonin

    d. dopamine
    e. none of above

Answer:

15. The smallest, simplest pathway to receive and process a stimulus is the

    a. reflex
    b. CNS
    c. ANS

    d. neuroglia
    e. none of above

Answer:

16. Some of the most commonly abused drugs are

    a. steroids
    b. depressants
    c. stimulants

    d. hallucinogens
    e. all of above

Answer:

17. Ganglia are found

    a. in the brain
    b. in the cortex
    c. in a tract

    d. outside the brain
    e. none of above

Answer:

18. Gray matter is found in the

    a. cortex
    b. myelin
    c. neuroglia

    d. nerve tracts
    e. none of above

Answer:

19. The tough mother is the

    a. pia mater
    b. dura mater
    c. spider layer

    d. arachnoid mater
    e. posterior root

Answer:

20. The layer containing numerous blood vessels and nerves is the

    a. pia mater
    b. spider layer
    c. dura mater

    d. arachnoid mater
    e. subdural space

Answer:

21. The spider layer is the

    a. pia mater
    b. dura mater
    c. subdural space

    d. arachnoid mater
    e. epidural space

Answer:

22. Serous fluid is found in the

    a. pia mater
    b. dura mater
    c. arachnoid mater

    d. subdural space
    e. epidural space

Answer:

23. Spinal taps are done in which region of the spine?

    a. cervical
    b. thoracic
    c. lumbar

    d. sacral
    e. coccyx

Answer:

24. Meninges are separated from the vertebrae by the

    a. subdural space
    b. spider layer
    c. epidural space

    d. pia mater
    e. subarachnoid space

Answer:

25. The functions of the spinal cord include

    a. reflex/respiration
    b. reflex/emotion
    c. reflex/cogitation

    d. reflex/conveyance
    e. reflex/protection

Answer:

26. The enzyme that breaks down acetylcholine is

    a. an anabolic steroid
    b. sodium
    c. acetylcholinesterase

    d. dopamine
    e. serotonin

Answer:

27. Heartbeat rate, digestion, and breathing rates are controlled and maintained by reflexes concerned with ___ processes.

    a. respiratory
    b. involuntary
    c. cognitive

    d. cortical
    e. somatic

Answer:

28. How many pairs of spinal nerves are there?

    a. 5
    b. 12
    c. 23

    d. 31
    e. 40

Answer:

CHAPTER 11

The Nervous System: The Brain, Cranial Nerves, Autonomic Nervous System, and the Special Senses

OBJECTIVES

After studying this chapter, you should be able to:

1. List the principal parts of the brain.
2. Name the functions of the cerebrospinal fluid.
3. List the principal functions of the major parts of the brain.
4. List the 12 cranial nerves and their functions.
5. Name the parts of the autonomic nervous system and describe how it functions.
6. Describe the basic anatomy of the sense organs and explain how they function.

ACTIVITIES

A. Completion

Fill in the blank spaces with the correct term.

1. The brain is protected by the ___ ___ and the ___.
2. The brain weighs ___ ___.
3. The three cranial meninges are the ___ mater, the ___ mater, and the ___ mater.
4. The bridge of nerve fibers connecting the two sides of the brain is the ___ ___.

NAME: _____   DATE: _____

5. The third and fourth ventricles are connected by the ___ ___.

6. The area contained within the medulla having dispersed gray matter is the ___ ___.

7. The midbrain contains the ___ ___ ___.

8. The diencephalon is divided into the ___ and the ___.

9. The optic tracts and optic chiasma are within the ___.

10. The mammillary bodies are involved in ___ and ___ ___.

11. The superior part of the diencephalon that plays a role in conscious recognition of pain is the ___.

12. The surface of the cerebrum made up of gray matter is known as the ___ ___.

13. The right and left hemispheres of the brain are separated by the ___ ___.

14. The ___ lobe is behind the frontal lobe.

15. Deep within the lateral sulcus is the ___.

16. The second largest portion of the brain is the ___.

17. The autonomic nervous system, a subdivision of the peripheral nervous system, has two parts; they are the ___ and the ___.

18. There are ___ pairs of cranial nerves.

19. The sense of smell is the ___ sense.

20. In the cilia that detect odors are ___.

21. The ___ ___ actually function as the receptors of the taste cells.

22. There are four major taste sensations; they are ___, ___, ___, and ___.

23. The black layer of the eye, which absorbs light, is the ___.

24. The portion of the eye that regulates the amount of light that enters the eye is the ___.

25. The area producing the sharpest vision is the ___ ___.

26. The two openings on the medial side of the middle ear are ___ ___ and the ___ ___.

27. The vestibule and the semicircular canals are involved in ___.

28. Inflammation of brain tissue is called ___.

29. ___ ___ is characterized by tremors of the hand.

30. Brain damage during brain development or the birth process can result in ___ ___.

31. ___ can be corrected by the use of reading glasses.

32. ___ ___ is caused by a stimulation of the semicircular canals of the inner ear.

33. Opacity of the lens is also known as ___.

B. Matching

Match the term on the right with the definition on the left.

_____ 34. protect the brain

_____ 35. cavities within the brain

_____ 36. shock absorber for the CNS

_____ 37. contains ascending and descending tracts

_____ 38. bridge brain and spinal cord

a. sulci

b. thalamus

c. papillae

d. otitis media

e. corpus callosum

_____ 39. superior part of the diencephalon

_____ 40. mesencephalon

_____ 41. groove in the brain

_____ 42. connects cerebral hemispheres

_____ 43. deep in the lateral sulcus

_____ 44. shaped like a butterfly

_____ 45. fight or flight

_____ 46. taste buds

_____ 47. transparent front of the eye

_____ 48. eye liquid

_____ 49. hammer

_____ 50. stirrup

_____ 51. tympanic membrane

_____ 52. from the ear to the pharynx

_____ 53. middle ear infection

f. cornea

g. stapes

h. aqueous humor

i. cerebrospinal fluid

j. pons varolii

k. eustachian tube

l. cerebellum

m. cranial meninges

n. malleus

o. medulla oblongata

p. sympathetic ANS

q. midbrain

r. insula

s. ventricles

t. eardrum

C. Key Terms

Use the text to look up the following terms. Write the definition or explanation.

54. Abducens nerve VI:

_____

_____

55. Accessory nerve XI:

_____

_____

56. Aqueous humor:

_____

_____

57. Auditory/eustachian tube:

_____

_____

58. Auricle:

_____

_____

59. Autonomic nervous system:

_____

_____

60. Brainstem:

_____

_____

61. Cerebellum:

_____

_____

62. Cerebral aqueduct/aqueduct of Sylvius:

_____

_____

63. Cerebral cortex:

_____

_____

64. Cerebral hemispheres:

_____

_____

65. Cerebrum:

_____

_____

66. Cerumen:

_____

_____

67. Ceruminous glands:

_____

_____

68. Choroid:

_____

_____

69. Ciliary body:

_____

_____

70. Conjunctiva:

_____

_____

71. Conjunctivitis:

_____

_____

72. Cornea:

_____

_____

73. Corpus callosum:

_____

_____

74. Decussation of pyramids:

_____

_____

75. Diencephalon:

_____

_____

76. Dorsal tectum:

_____

_____

77. External auditory meatus:

_____

_____

78. Facial nerve VII:

_____

_____

79. Fovea centralis:

_____

_____

80. Frontal lobe:

_____

_____

81. Glaucoma:

_____

_____

82. Glossopharyngeal nerve IX:

_____

_____

83. Gyri:

_____

_____

84. Hypoglossal nerve XII:

_____

_____

85. Hypothalamus:

_____

_____

86. Incus:

_____

_____

87. Infundibulum:

_____

_____

88. Insula:

_____

_____

89. Interventricular foramen/foramen of Monroe:

_____

_____

90. Iris:

_____

_____

91. Lens:

_____

_____

92. Longitudinal fissure:

_____

_____

93. Malleus:

_____

_____

94. Mammillary bodies:

_____

_____

95. Medulla oblongata:

_____

_____

96. Midbrain/mesencephalon:

_____

_____

97. Occipital lobe:

_____

_____

98. Oculomotor nerve III:

_____

_____

99. Olfactory nerve I:

_____

_____

100. Olfactory sense:

_____

_____

101. Optic chiasma:

_____

_____

102. Optic disk:

_____

_____

103. Optic nerve II:

_____

_____

104. Optic tracts:

_____

_____

105. Oval window:

_____

_____

106. Papillae:

_____

_____

107. Parasympathetic division:

_____

_____

108. Parietal lobe:

_____

_____

109. Parkinson's disease:

_____

_____

110. Pineal gland:

_____

_____

111. Pituitary gland:

_____

_____

112. Pons varolii:

_____

_____

113. Pupil:

_____

_____

114. Reticular formation:

_____

_____

115. Retina:

_____

_____

116. Rhodopsin:

_____

_____

117. Round window:

_____

_____

118. Sclera:

_____

_____

119. Stapes:

_____

_____

120. Sulci:

_____

_____

121. Sympathetic division:

_____

_____

122. Taste buds:

_____

_____

123. Taste cells:

_____

_____

124. Temporal lobe:

_____

_____

125. Thalamus:

_____

_____

126. Trigeminal nerve V:

_____

_____

127. Trochlear nerve IV:

_____

_____

128. Tympanic membrane:

_____

_____

129. Vagus nerve X:

_____

_____

130. Ventral cerebral peduncles:

_____

_____

131. Ventricles:

_____

_____

132. Vestibulocochlear nerve VIII:

_____

_____

133. Vitreous humor:

_____

_____

D. Labeling Exercise

134. Label the parts of the ear as indicated in Figure 11-1.

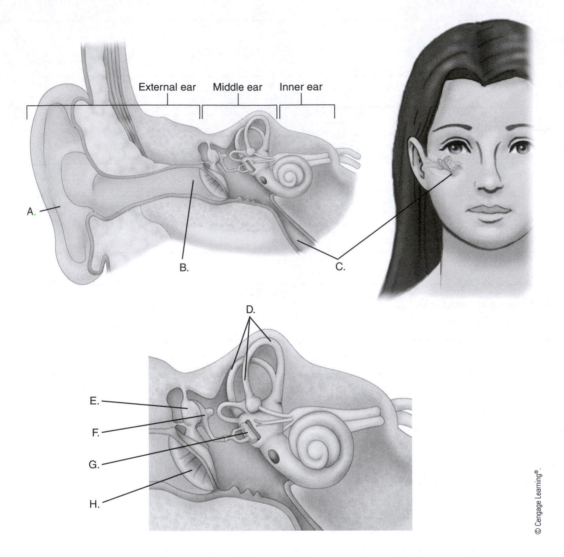

Figure 11-1

A. _____   E. _____

B. _____   F. _____

C. _____   G. _____

D. _____   H. _____

135. Label the parts of the eye as indicated in Figure 11-2.

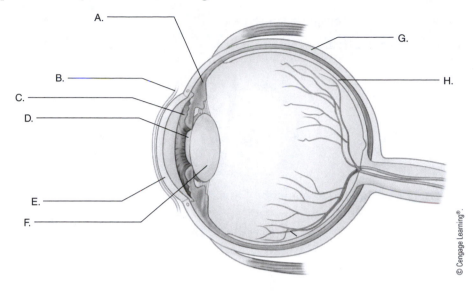

Figure 11-2

A. _____   E. _____

B. _____   F. _____

C. _____   G. _____

D. _____   H. _____

E. Coloring Exercise

136. Using Figure 11-3, color the frontal lobe green, the temporal lobe yellow, the parietal lobe blue, the occipital lobe red, the cerebellum brown, and the brain stem tan.

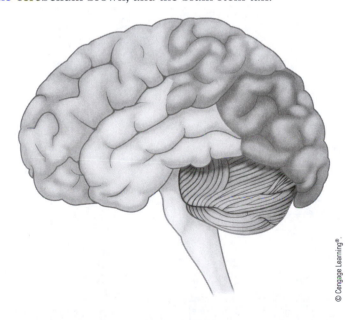

Figure 11-3

F. Critical Thinking

Answer the following questions in complete sentences.

137. Explain the mechanism of the fight-or-flight response.

138. What is the importance of the hypothalamus?

139. How would damage to the cerebellum affect the body?

140. How can the common cold affect the sense of taste?

141. How does flying in an airplane affect hearing?

142. Why should children not go to school when they have "pinkeye"?

143. Why do some middle-aged people have to get reading glasses?

144. What would be a possible treatment for glaucoma?

145. Identify age-related changes in the nervous system. Briefly explain the effects these changes have on older adults.

146. Of the career options associated with the nervous system, select the one that is most interesting to you. Tell why you consider this option as a potential career.

147. Distinguish between a psychiatrist and a psychologist.

G. Crossword Puzzle

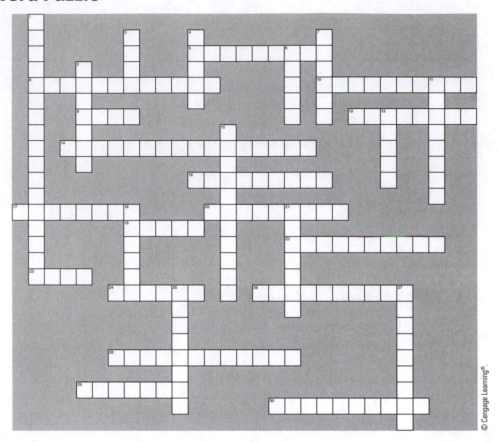

Complete the crossword puzzle using the following clues.

ACROSS

5. Nerve that controls head movements
8. Diencephalon part attached to the pituitary
9. Eyeball's colored part
10. Decrease in near vision
12. Seizures
14. Nerve that senses taste
16. Smallest of the cranial nerves
17. Relays sensory impulses
19. Retina cells that produce color
20. Nerve that controls smell
22. Largest of the cranial nerves
23. Retina cells very sensitive to light
24. Nerve that controls tear glands
26. Nerve that controls eyelid movement
28. Surrounds the third ventricle
29. Earwax
30. Headache

DOWN

1. Nerve that controls balance and hearing
2. Outer part of the ear
3. Brain folds
4. Nerve that conveys sensation in the larynx
6. Nerve that conveys vision impulses
7. Nearsightedness
11. Elevations of the tongue
13. Anvil
15. Nerve that controls swallowing
18. Eye's outermost layer
21. Lockjaw
25. Nerve that controls eyeball movement
27. Rod pigment

CHAPTER QUIZ

1. The disease that produces convulsive seizures is

   a. epilepsy
   b. cerebral palsy
   c. otitis media

   d. tetanus
   e. encephalitis

Answer:

2. The disease that produces infection in the middle ear is

   a. epilepsy
   b. cerebral palsy
   c. otitis media

   d. tetanus
   e. encephalitis

Answer:

3. The disease that produces defective muscular coordination is

   a. epilepsy
   b. cerebral palsy
   c. otitis media

   d. tetanus
   e. encephalitis

Answer:

4. Farsightedness is

   a. myopia
   b. hyperopia
   c. presbyopia

   d. glaucoma
   e. amblyopia

Answer:

5. An accommodation disease of aging is

   a. myopia
   b. hyperopia
   c. presbyopia

   d. glaucoma
   e. amblyopia

Answer:

6. A disease that causes destruction of the retina is

   a. myopia
   b. hyperopia
   c. presbyopia

   d. glaucoma
   e. amblyopia

Answer:

7. Nearsightedness is

   a. myopia
   b. hyperopia
   c. presbyopia

   d. glaucoma
   e. amblyopia

Answer:

8. The part of the ear allowing for pressure equalization is the

   a. stapes
   b. vestibule
   c. auricle

   d. tympanum
   e. eustachian tube

Answer:

9. The part of the ear allowing for balance is the

   a. stapes
   b. vestibule
   c. auricle

   d. tympanum
   e. eustachian tube

Answer:

10. The part of the ear acting like a drum head is the

   a. stapes
   b. vestibule
   c. auricle

   d. tympanic membrane
   e. eustachian tube

Answer:

11. Night blindness can be caused by a deficiency of

   a. vitamin A
   b. vitamin D
   c. vitamin K

   d. vitamin B
   e. vitamin E

Answer:

12. The ability to see color is due to

   a. rods
   b. choroid
   c. cones

   d. sclera
   e. lens

Answer:

13. The white, outermost layer of the eye is the

   a. pupil
   b. choroid
   c. retina

   d. sclera
   e. lens

Answer:

14. The cells of the retina that synapse with ganglia cells are

   a. unipolar
   b. bipolar
   c. conical

   d. multipolar
   e. photoreceptors

Answer:

15. Glaucoma is caused by a defect of the

   a. sclera
   b. vitreous humor
   c. aqueous humor

   d. lens
   e. choroid

Answer:

16. Rhodopsin is found in the

    a. rods   d. choroid
    b. sclera   e. lens
    c. cones

Answer:

17. The actual taste function is found on the

    a. papillae   d. taste hairs
    b. salivary glands   e. epithelial cells
    c. taste pores

Answer:

18. Chemoreceptors are used in the sense of

    a. taste   d. hearing
    b. sight   e. touch
    c. smell

Answer:

19. The cranial nerves number

    a. 6   d. 36
    b. 12   e. 48
    c. 24

Answer:

20. The neurotransmitter associated with the parasympathetic system is

    a. epinephrine   d. serotonin
    b. adrenaline   e. acetylcholine
    c. norepinephrine

Answer:

21. Which of the following is NOT a function of the cerebellum?

    a. reflex   d. balance
    b. coordination   e. movement
    c. posture

Answer:

22. Which lobe of the cerebrum evaluates hearing input?

    a. parietal   d. occipital
    b. frontal   e. none of the above
    c. temporal

Answer:

23. Which lobe of the cerebrum is involved in visual input?

    a. parietal   d. occipital
    b. frontal   e. none of the above
    c. temporal

Answer:

24. Which lobe of the cerebrum is involved in evaluating sensory information?

    a. parietal
    b. frontal
    c. temporal
    d. occipital
    e. none of the above

Answer:

25. Which lobe of the cerebrum controls moods, aggression, and motivation?

    a. parietal
    b. frontal
    c. temporal
    d. occipital
    e. none of the above

Answer:

26. Each hemisphere has folds called

    a. gyri
    b. sulci
    c. fissures
    d. lobes
    e. none of the above

Answer:

27. The mind controlling the body phenomenon is located in the

    a. thalamus
    b. hypothalamus
    c. midbrain
    d. cerebellum
    e. none of the above

Answer:

28. The ventral cerebral peduncles are contained in the

    a. cerebellum
    b. cerebrum
    c. medulla oblongata
    d. midbrain
    e. none of the above

Answer:

29. The foramen of Monroe connects

    a. sulci
    b. gyri
    c. ventricles
    d. lobes
    e. none of the above

Answer:

30. Which of the following is an area of the brainstem?

    a. medulla oblongata
    b. thalamus
    c. cerebellum
    d. corpus callosum
    e. none of the above

Answer:

31. What is the outermost layer of the cranial meninges?

    a. pia mater
    b. arachnoid mater
    c. occipital lobe
    d. dura mater
    e. corpus callosum

Answer:

32. The part of the epithalamus that secretes melatonin is the

    a. pineal gland
    b. pituitary gland
    c. mammillary body
    d. thalamus
    e. optic chiasma

Answer:

33. The colored part of the eye that consists of smooth muscle surrounding the pupil is the

    a. cornea
    b. sclera
    c. choroid
    d. iris
    e. vitreous humor

Answer:

The Endocrine System

After studying this chapter, you should be able to:

1. List the functions of hormones.

2. Classify hormones into their major chemical categories.

3. Describe how the hypothalamus of the brain controls the endocrine system.

4. Name the endocrine glands and state where they are located.

5. List the major hormones and their effects on the body.

6. Discuss some of the major diseases of the endocrine system and their causes.

ACTIVITIES

A. Completion

Fill in the blank spaces with the correct term.

1. The hypothalamus sends directions to the pituitary gland by ___ ___.

2. Endocrine glands are ductless glands. This means they secrete their hormones directly into the ___.

3. Negative feedback means that when a hormone reaches a certain level, the gland's secretion is ___.

4. Hormones can be classified into ___ categories.

5. The simplest group of hormones is the modified ___ ___.

6. The second category of hormones is the ___ hormones.

7. ___ are the third kind of hormones.

8. Steroid hormones are soluble in ___.

NAME: _____   DATE: _____

9. Because they cannot diffuse across the intestinal lining, protein and modified amino acid hormones like insulin must be ___.

10. Anabolic steroids are variants of ___.

11. Athletes use anabolic steroids to build ___ ___.

12. The chemical signals of the hypothalamus are called ___ ___ and ___ ___.

13. The pituitary gland is also called the ___.

14. The pituitary gland has two lobes, the ___ and the ___ lobes.

15. The larger of the lobes produces ___ hormones.

16. TSH stimulates the ___ gland to produce its hormone.

17. MSH increases the production of melanin and this ___ the skin.

18. Luteinizing hormone stimulates ___ in the female.

19. ADH inhibits the body from excreting ___.

20. Oxytocin stimulates contraction of the uterus and also stimulates ___.

21. A goiter is an enlarged ___ gland.

22. To properly function, the thyroid gland must have ___.

23. The parathyroid glands consist of ___ cells and ___ cells.

24. The hormone from the parathyroid glands functions to balance ___ levels in the body.

25. The adrenal medulla secretes ___; the adrenal cortex secretes a number of hormones, the most important of which is ___.

26. The middle layer of the adrenal cortex secretes ___, which is also known as ___.

27. The sex hormones secreted by the inner layer of the adrenal cortex are ___.

28. The islets of Langerhans are located on the ___, and they produce the hormones ___ and ___.

29. Glycosuria is a condition of elevated sugar in the ___.

30. The thymus gland is important in the development of ___.

31. ___ syndrome is caused by a long-term excessive production of cortisol.

32. Adrenogenital syndrome occurs due to excessive secretion of androgens from the ___ ___.

33. ___ affective disorder produces a type of depression.

B. Matching

Match the term on the right with the definition on the left.

____ 34. secretes into blood   a. adrenals

____ 35. have ducts   b. thyroxine

____ 36. simplest hormones   c. pituitary gland

____ 37. stimulates or inhibits hormone release   d. cortisol

____ 38. controls many glands   e. oxytocin

____ 39. stimulates cell metabolism   f. parathormone

____ 40. darkens the skin   g. prolactin

____ 41. maintains progesterone during pregnancy   h. Graves disease

_____ 42. maintains water balance

_____ 43. ADH deficiency

_____ 44. stimulates lactation

_____ 45. enlarged thyroid

_____ 46. contains four iodine atoms

_____ 47. hyperthyroidism

_____ 48. lowers calcium level

_____ 49. inhibits osteoblasts

_____ 50. increases calcium absorption

_____ 51. atop kidneys

_____ 52. glucocorticoid hormone

_____ 53. regulates blood glucose

i. vitamin D

j. MSH

k. modified amino acids

l. glucagon

m. calcitonin

n. diabetes insipidus

o. exocrine

p. vasopressin

q. neurosecretion

r. goiter

s. growth hormone

t. ductless glands

C. Key Terms

Use the text to look up the following terms. Write the definition or explanation.

54. Acidosis:

_____

_____

55. Addison's disease:

_____

_____

56. Adrenal cortex:

_____

_____

57. Adrenal glands/suprarenal glands:

_____

_____

58. Adrenal medulla:

_____

_____

59. Adrenaline/epinephrine:

_____

_____

60. Adrenocorticotropic hormone/ACTH:

_____

_____

61. Adrenogenital syndrome:

_____

_____

62. Aldosterone:

_____

_____

63. Aldosteronism:

_____

_____

64. Alpha cells:

_____

_____

65. Androgens:

_____

_____

66. Antidiuretic hormone/ADH/vasopressin:

_____

_____

67. Beta cells:

_____

_____

68. Calcitonin:

_____

_____

69. Chief cells:

_____

_____

70. Cortisol/hydrocortisone:

_____

_____

71. Cortisone:

_____

_____

72. Cretinism:

_____

_____

73. Cushing's syndrome:

_____

_____

74. Diabetes insipidus:

_____

_____

75. Diabetes mellitus:

_____

_____

76. Endocrine glands:

_____

_____

77. Estrogen:

_____

_____

78. Exophthalmia:

_____

_____

79. Follicle-stimulating hormone (FSH):

_____

_____

80. Glucagon:

_____

_____

81. Glycosuria:

_____

_____

82. Goiter:

_____

_____

83. Graves' disease:

_____

_____

84. Growth hormone:

_____

_____

85. Homeostasis:

_____

_____

86. Hormones:

_____

_____

87. Hyperglycemia:

_____

_____

88. Hyperparathyroidism:

_____

_____

89. Hyperthyroidism:

_____

_____

90. Hypoparathyroidism:

_____

_____

91. Hypophysis:

_____

_____

92. Hypothalamus:

_____

_____

93. Hypothyroidism:

_____

_____

94. Infundibulum:

_____

_____

95. Insulin:

_____

_____

96. Lactogenic hormone (LTH)/Prolactin:

_____

_____

97. Luteinizing hormone (LH):

_____

_____

98. Melanocyte-stimulating hormone (MSH):

_____

_____

99. Melatonin:

_____

_____

100. Myxedema:

_____

_____

101. Negative feedback system:

_____

_____

102. Noradrenaline/norepinephrine:

_____

_____

103. Ovaries:

_____

_____

104. Oxyphil cells:

_____

_____

105. Oxytocin (OT):

_____

_____

106. Pancreatic islets/islets of Langerhans:

_____

_____

107. Parathyroid glands:

_____

_____

108. Parathyroid hormone/ parathormone (PTH):

_____

_____

109. Pineal gland/body:

_____

_____

110. Pituitary gland/hypophysis:

_____

_____

111. Polydipsia:

_____

_____

112. Polyphagia:

_____

_____

113. Polyuria:

_____

_____

114. Progesterone:

_____

_____

115. Releasing hormones:

_____

_____

116. Releasing inhibitory hormones:

_____

_____

117. Seasonal affective disorder:

_____

_____

118. Serotonin:

_____

_____

119. Stress:

_____

_____

120. Testes:

_____

_____

121. Testosterone:

_____

_____

122. Thymosin:

_____

_____

123. Thymus gland:

_____

_____

124. Thyroid gland:

_____

_____

125. Thyroid-stimulating hormone (TSH):

_____

_____

126. Thyroxine or tetraiodothyronine (T_4):

_____

_____

127. Triiodothyronine (T_3):

_____

_____

D. Labeling Exercise

128. Label the parathyroid glands and their cellular components as indicated in Figure 12-1.

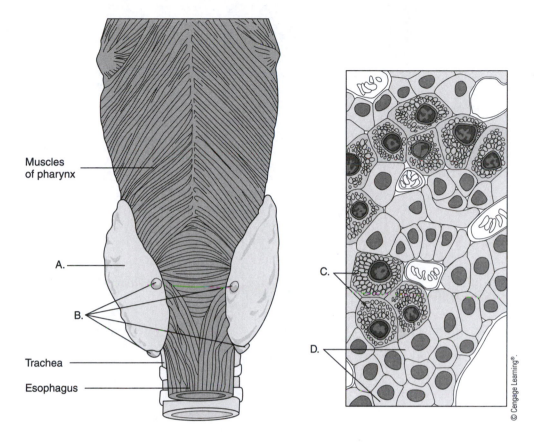

Figure 12-1

A. _____

B. _____

C. _____

D. _____

129. Label the endocrine glands as indicated in Figure 12-2.

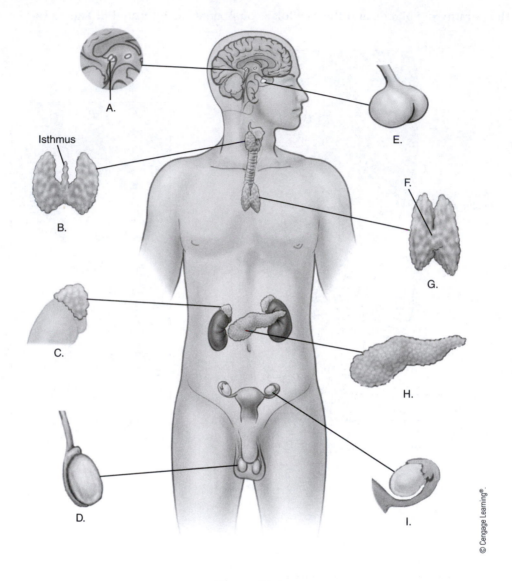

Figure 12-2

A. _____   F. _____

B. _____   G. _____

C. _____   H. _____

D. _____   I. _____

E. _____   J. _____

E. Coloring Exercise

130. Using Figure 12-3, color the corpus callosum red, the thalamus blue, the pineal gland green, the pituitary gland yellow, and the hypothalamus brown.

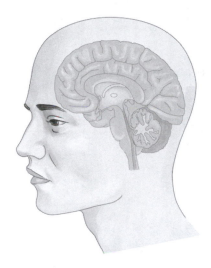 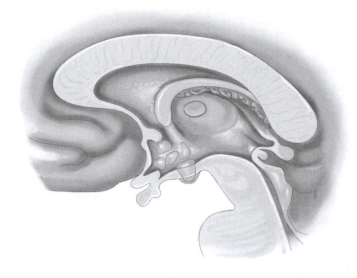

© Cengage Learning®

Figure 12-3

F. Critical Thinking

Answer the following questions in complete sentences.

131. Why must hormones like insulin and oxytocin be injected?

132. Explain some of the dangers associated with overuse of anabolic steroids.

133. Why does excess secretion of growth hormone in childhood produce gigantism and in adulthood acromegaly?

134. Why are goiters much less common today than 100 years ago?

135. Explain the difference between the effects of hypothyroidism in adults and in children.

136. Explain the effects of hypoparathyroidism.

137. Differentiate between diabetes mellitus type 1 and type 2.

138. Identify age-related changes to the endocrine system and one effective strategy for offsetting these changes.

139. Evaluate your interest and abilities for one of these career paths: nuclear medicine technologist, endocrinologist, or diabetes dietician.

G. Crossword Puzzle

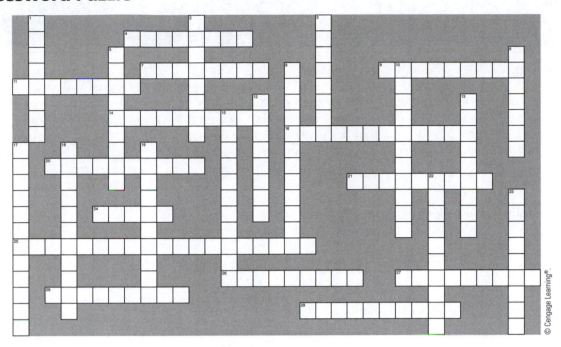

Complete the crossword puzzle using the following clues.

ACROSS

4. Stimulates uterine contraction
7. Hormone producing T lymphocytes
9. Pineal gland hormone
11. Secreted from the adrenal cortex
14. Enlarged hands and feet
16. Male sex hormone
20. Secreted by the thyroid gland
21. Adrenal sex hormones
24. Route for hormone transport
25. Bones become soft
26. Ductless glands
27. Stimulated by luteinizing hormone
28. Master gland of endocrine system
29. Pituitary gland

DOWN

1. Female sex hormone
2. Control the body's internal environment
3. Low blood pH
5. Stimulates milk production
6. Secreted by pancreatic islets
8. Inferior diencephalon
10. Fight-or-flight hormone
12. Adult hypothyroidism condition
13. Children's hypothyroidism
15. Regulates sodium reabsorption
17. Bulging eyes
18. Antidiuretic hormone
19. Intense food craving
22. Excess sugar in urine
23. Acts as vasoconstrictor

CASE STUDY

Isabella, a 48-year-old woman, is seeing a health care provider at her HMO. The care provider notes that Isabella's eyes are protruding, and her hands have a slight tremor. Isabella states that she has been feeling nervous, anxious, and extremely exhausted. She has also been experiencing heart palpitations. In addition, she says that she lost 10 pounds over the last two weeks without dieting. The care provider examines Isabella's neck and finds that her thyroid gland is enlarged. Based on these findings, the care provider refers Isabella to a specialist for further evaluation.

QUESTIONS

1. What endocrine disorder might Isabella have?

2. Elevations of which hormones are responsible for causing this disorder?

3. What type of medical specialist should Isabella see for further evaluation?

4. How is this condition treated?

CHAPTER QUIZ

1. The gland crucial to the immune system is the

   a. pituitary   d. adrenal
   b. thymus   e. pineal
   c. thyroid

Answer:

2. The gland responsible for the secretion of melatonin is the

   a. pituitary   d. adrenal
   b. thymus   e. pineal
   c. thyroid

Answer:

3. The gland that secretes cortisol is the

   a. pituitary   d. adrenal
   b. thymus   e. pineal
   c. thyroid

Answer:

4. The secretion that regulates the blood sugar level is

   a. cortisol
   b. thyroxin
   c. glucagon
   d. melatonin
   e. none of the above

Answer:

5. A low blood sugar level can cause

   a. acidosis
   b. pancreatitis
   c. hypothyroidism
   d. goiter
   e. none of the above

Answer:

6. Epinephrine is secreted by the

   a. pituitary
   b. thyroid
   c. thymus
   d. pancreas
   e. none of the above

Answer:

7. Vitamin D increases the absorption of

   a. sodium
   b. calcium
   c. chlorine
   d. potassium
   e. none of the above

Answer:

8. Which of the following glands needs iodine to function correctly?

   a. thymus
   b. pituitary
   c. thyroid
   d. adrenal
   e. none of the above

Answer:

9. ADH helps maintain proper water balance in the body. It is also called

   a. vasopressin
   b. adrenaline
   c. thymosin
   d. oxytocin
   e. none of the above

Answer:

10. The hormone that stimulates ovary follicle development and sperm cell production is

   a. FSH
   b. MSH
   c. LH
   d. TSH
   e. none of the above

Answer:

11. The master gland is controlled by the

   a. pituitary
   b. thalamus
   c. hypothalamus
   d. cerebellum
   e. none of the above

Answer:

12. The hormones that can diffuse across cell membranes are the

    a. proteins
    b. steroids
    c. amino acids

    d. oxytocin
    e. none of the above

Answer:

13. Which of the following is NOT a function of hormones?

    a. growth
    b. reproduction
    c. behavior patterns

    d. maturation
    e. metabolism

Answer:

14. Which of the following organs controls water levels and electrolyte balance?

    a. pancreas
    b. liver
    c. kidneys

    d. heart
    e. none of the above

Answer:

15. The production of T lymphocytes is done in the

    a. thyroid
    b. pituitary
    c. parathyroid

    d. thymus
    e. none of the above

Answer:

16. Glycogen is stored for use between meals. It is stored in which organ?

    a. pancreas
    b. liver
    c. kidneys

    d. heart
    e. none of the above

Answer:

17. The functions of the reproductive system are inhibited by

    a. thymosin
    b. melatonin
    c. renin

    d. thyroxine
    e. none of the above

Answer:

18. The pineal gland secretes which two substances?

    a. melatonin/serotonin
    b. thyroxine/thymosin
    c. estrogen/progesterone

    d. ADH/oxytocin
    e. none of the above

Answer:

19. Polyuria, polydipsia, and polyphagia are associated with

    a. gigantism
    b. cretinism
    c. acromegaly

    d. diabetes
    e. none of the above

Answer:

20. If blood glucose decreases excessively, fatty acids and what are released to cause acidosis?

    a. proteins
    b. sugar
    c. ketones

    d. steroids
    e. none of the above

Answer:

21. Pancreatic juice is produced by

    a. acini cells
    b. alpha cells
    c. beta cells

    d. red cells
    e. none of the above

Answer:

22. Insulin is produced by

    a. acini cells
    b. alpha cells
    c. beta cells

    d. red cells
    e. none of the above

Answer:

23. Glucagon is produced by the

    a. acini cells
    b. alpha cells
    c. beta cells

    d. red cells
    e. none of the above

Answer:

24. Androgens are produced by the

    a. acini cells
    b. alpha cells
    c. beta cells

    d. red cells
    e. none of the above

Answer:

25. Overproduction of hormones by the adrenal cortex can lead to

    a. Addison's disease
    b. Graves' disease
    c. Cushing's syndrome

    d. cretinism
    e. none of the above

Answer:

26. A bronzing of the skin is a symptom of which disease?

    a. Addison's disease
    b. Graves' disease
    c. Cushing's syndrome

    d. cretinism
    e. none of the above

Answer:

27. The gland sitting atop the kidney is the

    a. pituitary
    b. adrenal
    c. thymus

    d. thyroid
    e. none of the above

Answer:

28. Which of the following hormones is secreted by the thyroid gland?

    a. serotonin
    b. oxytocin
    c. calcitonin

    d. cortisol
    e. melatonin

Answer:

29. Which of the following is a disease of the thyroid gland?

    a. Cushing's syndrome
    b. acromegaly
    c. Addison's disease

    d. goiter
    e. none of the above

Answer:

30. Which of the following stimulates milk production?

    a. FSH
    b. LTH
    c. MSH

    d. LH
    e. none of the above

Answer:

31. Which hormone stimulates the thyroid gland to produce its own hormone?

    a. TSH
    b. FSH
    c. MSH

    d. LH
    e. calcitonin

Answer:

32. What makes up the bulk of the adrenal gland?

    a. adrenal medulla
    b. adrenal cortex
    c. Bowman's capsule

    d. skeletal muscle
    e. kidney

Answer:

33. Thymosin causes the production of which of the following?

    a. white blood cells
    b. FSH
    c. thyroid hormone

    d. platelets
    e. none of the above

Answer:

The Blood

OBJECTIVES

After studying this chapter, you should be able to:

1. Describe the functions of blood.
2. Classify the different types of blood cells.
3. Describe the anatomy of erythrocytes relative to their function.
4. Compare the functions of the different leukocytes.
5. Explain how and where blood cells are formed.
6. Explain the clotting mechanism.
7. Name the different blood groups.

ACTIVITIES

A. Completion

Fill in the blank spaces with the correct term.

1. Platelets are also called ___.
2. The white cells are the ___ and the red cells are the ___.
3. Blood transports oxygen from the lungs and ___ ___ to the lungs.
4. The regulation of water by the blood plays a role in the process of ___.
5. Neutrophils, eosinophils, and basophils are the ___ leukocytes.
6. Of the three proteins in plasma, ___ is the one that plays a role in maintaining water balance.
7. ___ carries hormones to target organs.
8. Blood cell formation occurs in ___ ___.

NAME: _____   DATE: _____

9. Lymphocytes and monocytes are produced in certain ___ tissue.

10. Undifferentiated mesenchymal cells are called ___.

11. Some stem cells will become ___, and these mature into erythrocytes.

12. Red blood cells do not have a(n) ___.

13. Heme contains the element ___.

14. Although leukocytes have a nucleus, they do not have any ___.

15. Leukocytes clean up foreign bodies by ___.

16. The destruction of certain bacteria is accomplished by the enzyme ___.

17. After they leave the blood and enter tissues, ___ increase in size.

18. Disk-shaped cellular fragments with a nucleus are the ___.

19. In the first stage of clotting, ___ is released.

20. In the second stage of clotting, prothrombin is converted to ___.

21. The formation of the clot is a result of the production of ___.

22. After the clot forms, the plasma remaining is called ___.

23. After tissue repair, fibrinolysis occurs; this is a(n) ___ of the blood clot.

24. Clotting in an unbroken vessel is called ___.

25. A piece of a thrombus that breaks off is a(n) ___.

26. Antigens on the red blood cell membrane are the basis of blood ___.

27. The universal donor is a person with blood type ___.

28. A genetically inherited blood clotting disease is ___.

29. Another hereditary blood disease causing suppressed hemoglobin production is ___.

30. Infectious mononucleosis is caused by the ___-___ virus.

31. A decrease in blood pressure caused by microorganisms and their toxins in the blood is referred to as ___ ___.

32. Hemolytic disease of the newborn is also called ___ ___.

33. Vitamin ___ plays a major role in many of the factors involved in blood clotting.

B. Matching

Match the term on the right with the definition on the left.

_____ 34. erythrocyte   a. leukocytes

_____ 35. thrombocyte   b. septicemia

_____ 36. 55% of blood   c. syneresis

_____ 37. granular leukocyte   d. hemolytic anemia

_____ 38. maintain osmotic pressure   e. embolus

_____ 39. vital role in clotting   f. plasma

_____ 40. stem cell   g. basophils

_____ 41. red pigment   h. platelets

_____ 42. no nuclei, no pigment

_____ 43. enzyme that destroys certain bacteria

_____ 44. involved in production of antibodies

_____ 45. production of prothrombin activation

_____ 46. clot retraction

_____ 47. dissolution of clot

_____ 48. piece of blood clot

_____ 49. clumping red blood cells

_____ 50. red cells destroyed

_____ 51. suppressed hemoglobin production

_____ 52. blood poisoning

_____ 53. produce serotonin

i. fibrinolysis

j. hematocytoblasts

k. fibrinogen

l. lymphocytes

m. thalassemia

n. albumin

o. red cell

p. thromboplastin

q. hemoglobin

r. lysozyme

s. agglutination

t. eosinophils

C. Key Terms

Use the text to look up the following terms. Write the definition or explanation.

54. ABO blood group:

_____

_____

55. Agglutination:

_____

_____

56. Albumin:

_____

_____

57. Basophils:

_____

_____

58. Clot:

_____

_____

59. Complement:

_____

_____

60. Embolism:

_____

_____

61. Embolus:

_____

_____

62. Eosinophils:

_____

_____

63. Erythroblastosis fetalis:

_____

_____

64. Erythrocytes:

_____

_____

65. Erythrocytosis:

_____

_____

66. Fibrin:

_____

_____

67. Fibrinogen:

_____

_____

68. Fibrinolysis:

_____

_____

69. Globin:

_____

_____

70. Globulins:

_____

_____

71. Hematopoiesis:

_____

_____

72. Heme:

_____

_____

73. Hemoglobin:

_____

_____

74. Hemophilia:

_____

_____

75. Infarction:

_____

_____

76. Leukocytes (WBCs):

_____

_____

77. Lymphocytes:

_____

_____

78. Lysozyme:

_____

_____

79. Macrophages:

_____

_____

80. Malaria:

_____

_____

81. Megakaryocytes:

_____

_____

82. Monocytes:

_____

_____

83. Myeloid tissue/red bone marrow:

_____

_____

84. Neutrophils:

_____

_____

85. Phagocytosis:

_____

_____

86. Plaque:

_____

_____

87. Plasma:

_____

_____

88. Prothrombin:

_____

_____

89. Rh blood group:

_____

_____

90. Stem cells/hematocytoblasts:

_____

_____

91. Syneresis:

_____

_____

92. Thrombin:

_____

_____

93. Thrombocytes/platelets:

_____

_____

94. Thrombocytopenia:

_____

_____

95. Thromboplastin:

_____

_____

96. Thrombosis:

_____

_____

97. Thrombus:

_____

_____

D. Labeling Exercise

98. Label the blood cells as indicated in Figure 13-1.

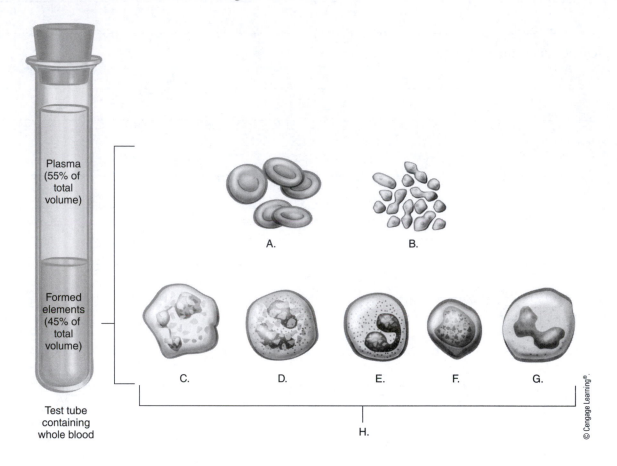

Figure 13-1

A. _____

B. _____

C. _____

D. _____

E. _____

F. _____

G. _____

H. _____

99. Label the various leukocytes as indicated in Figure 13-2.

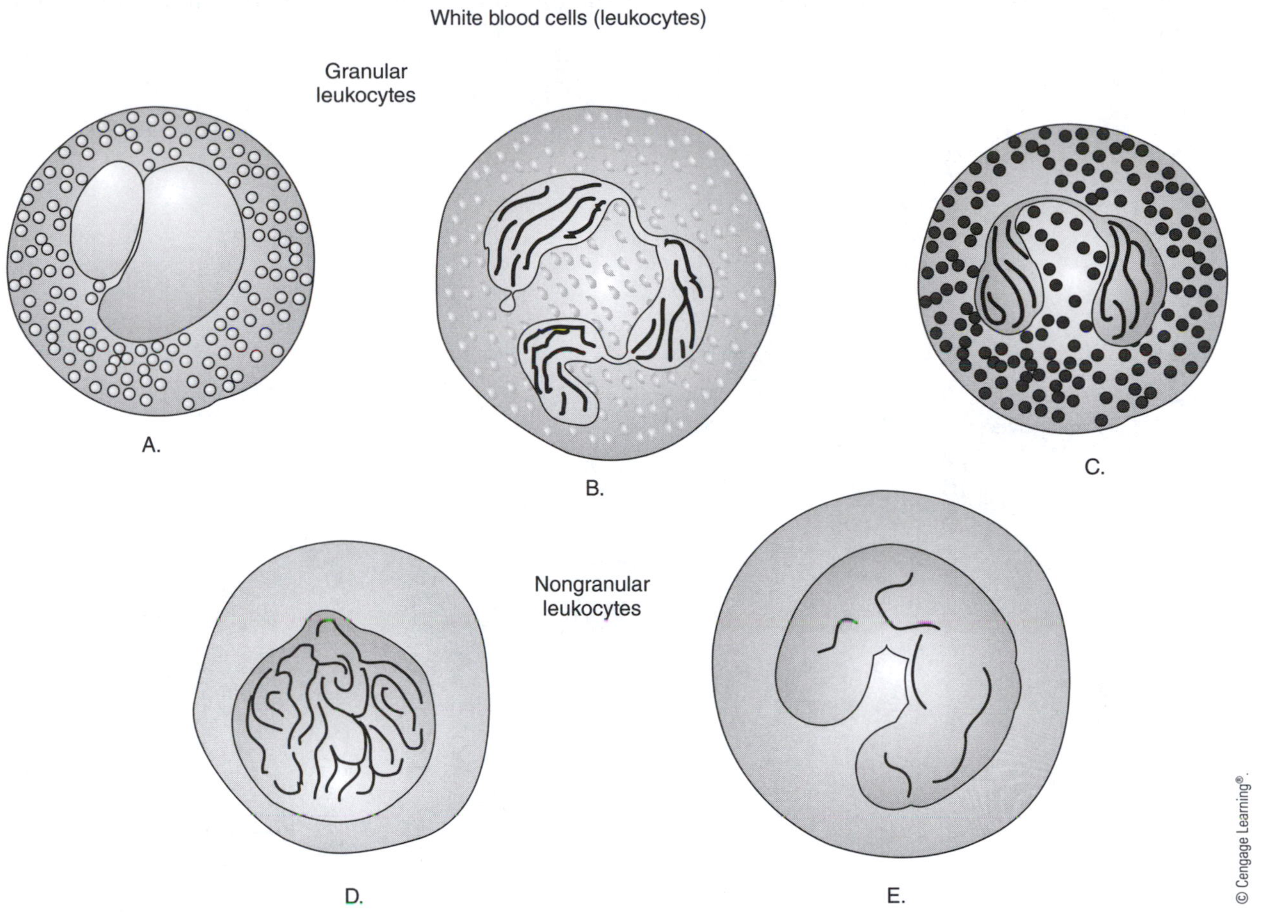

White blood cells (leukocytes)

Granular
leukocytes

A.

B.

C.

Nongranular
leukocytes

D.

E.

© Cengage Learning®

Figure 13-2

A. _____

B. _____

C. _____

D. _____

E. _____

E. Coloring Exercise

100. Using Figure 13-3, color the prothrombin yellow, the thromboplastin blue, the thrombin green, and the red cells red.

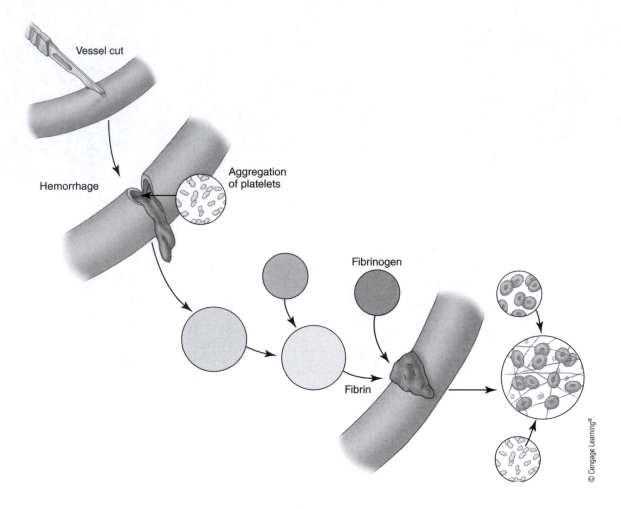

Vessel cut

Hemorrhage

Aggregation of platelets

Fibrinogen

Fibrin

© Cengage Learning®.

Figure 13-3

F. Critical Thinking

Answer the following questions in complete sentences.

101. How does blood help regulate body water content?

102. Explain hematopoiesis.

103. Describe the primary function of erythrocytes.

104. Explain the clotting mechanism process.

105. Explain blood typing.

106. How is erythroblastosis fetalis developed?

107. How does sickle-cell anemia work?

108. How can a clot cause death?

109. Explain the connection between the blood and vitamin K.

110. Explain why smoking may cause mental impairment.

111. Distinguish between a hematologist and an infectious disease specialist.

G. Crossword Puzzle

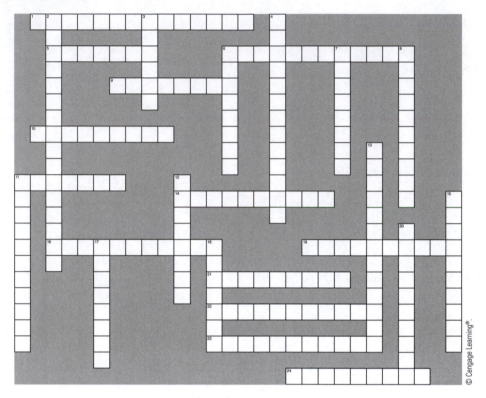

Complete the crossword puzzle using the following clues.

ACROSS

1. Prothrombin activator
5. *Anopheles* mosquito
6. Eating cells
9. Blood cancer
10. Clot retraction
11. Piece of blood clot
14. Red pigment
16. Suppressed hemoglobin production
19. Clotting disorder
21. Release heparin
22. Largest leukocytes
23. Most common leukocytes
24. Antibodies

DOWN

2. Stem cells
3. Cholesterol-containing mass
4. Red cells clump
6. Blood cells involved in clotting
7. Catalyst for fibrin
8. Blood poisoning
11. Combat irritants
12. Clot
13. Blood cell formation
15. Tissue killed
17. Bacteria destroyed in enzyme
18. Maintain osmotic pressure
20. Clotting

CASE STUDY

Frank, a 15-year-old high school student, tells his mother that he does not want to go to school today. Frank is complaining of a sore throat and swollen lymph nodes in his armpits. Frank's mother takes his temperature and notes he has a fever. Frank mentions that several classmates at school have recently had similar symptoms. That afternoon, Frank sees his health care provider who performs a physical examination and orders blood tests that include a complete white blood cell count.

QUESTIONS

1. What disorder might Frank have?

2. What is the major cause of this disorder?

3. Which type of leukocyte or white blood cell is altered and destroyed as a result of this condition?

4. What are the major symptoms of this problem?

CHAPTER QUIZ

1. The fluid part of the blood is called

   a. erythrocytes
   b. leukocytes
   c. thrombocytes
   d. plasma
   e. none of the above

Answer:

2. The amount of blood in the body is about

   a. 3–4 liters
   b. 6–7 liters
   c. 5–6 liters
   d. 4–5 liters
   e. none of the above

Answer:

3. Which of the following is NOT transported by the blood?

   a. water
   b. lymph
   c. oxygen
   d. carbon dioxide
   e. none of the above

Answer:

4. Which of the following parts of the blood play a role in temperature regulation?

    a. erythrocytes
    b. leukocytes
    c. water
    d. thrombocytes
    e. none of the above

Answer:

5. Which of the following is NOT a granular leukocyte?

    a. lymphocyte
    b. neutrophil
    c. eosinophil
    d. basophil
    e. none of the above

Answer:

6. The solid element of the blood responsible for clotting is the

    a. erythrocyte
    b. leukocyte
    c. thrombocyte
    d. albumin
    e. none of the above

Answer:

7. Which of the following is NOT present in the plasma?

    a. water
    b. fibrinogen
    c. albumin
    d. globulin
    e. none of the above

Answer:

8. Blood cells develop from all of the following EXCEPT

    a. mesenchymal cells
    b. stem cells
    c. hematocytoblasts
    d. lymphocytes
    e. none of the above

Answer:

9. Proerythroblasts eventually become

    a. erythrocytes
    b. leukocytes
    c. thrombocytes
    d. lymphoblasts
    e. none of the above

Answer:

10. Hemoglobin contains which of the following elements?

    a. sodium
    b. iron
    c. copper
    d. potassium
    e. none of the above

Answer:

11. The number of red blood cells in the female's body is

    a. 5.4 million
    b. 2.6 million
    c. 5–9 thousand
    d. 4–5 hundred thousand
    e. none of the above

Answer:

12. Neutrophils are the most common

    a. erythrocytes
    b. leukocytes
    c. thrombocytes
    d. lymphocytes
    e. none of the above

Answer:

13. Which of the following are phagocytic?

    a. neutrophils
    b. eosinophils
    c. basophils
    d. platelets
    e. none of the above

Answer:

14. Which of the following produce antihistamines?

    a. neutrophils
    b. eosinophils
    c. basophils
    d. platelets
    e. none of the above

Answer:

15. Which of the following produce heparin?

    a. neutrophils
    b. eosinophils
    c. basophils
    d. platelets
    e. none of the above

Answer:

16. Thrombocytes are produced in the red bone marrow from

    a. lymphocytes
    b. monocytes
    c. megakaryocytes
    d. macrophages
    e. none of the above

Answer:

17. Prothrombin is produced in which stage of coagulation?

    a. first
    b. second
    c. third
    d. fourth
    e. none of the above

Answer:

18. Fibrinogen is produced in which stage of coagulation?

    a. first
    b. second
    c. third
    d. fourth
    e. none of the above

Answer:

19. The material that actually forms the clot is

    a. prothrombin
    b. fibrinogen
    c. thrombin
    d. fibrin
    e. none of the above

Answer:

20. Clot retraction is called

   a. syneresis
   b. fibrinolysis
   c. hematopoiesis

   d. agglutination
   e. none of the above

Answer:

21. Clot dissolution is called

   a. syneresis
   b. fibrinolysis
   c. hematopoiesis

   d. agglutination
   e. none of the above

Answer:

22. Blood clumping is called

   a. syneresis
   b. fibrinolysis
   c. hematopoiesis

   d. agglutination
   e. none of the above

Answer:

23. A blood clot in the brain blocking a vessel is called a(n)

   a. coronary thrombosis
   b. cerebral thrombosis
   c. embolus

   d. pulmonary embolism
   e. none of the above

Answer:

24. Of the four blood groups, which of the following is the universal donor type?

   a. A
   b. B
   c. AB

   d. O
   e. none of the above

Answer:

25. Of the four blood groups, which of the following is the universal recipient type?

   a. A
   b. B
   c. AB

   d. O
   e. none of the above

Answer:

26. The hemolytic disease of the newborn is

   a. erythroblastosis fetalis
   b. hemophilia
   c. leukemia

   d. anemia
   e. none of the above

Answer:

27. The anemia caused by the abnormal shape of red blood cells is

   a. hemolytic
   b. leukemia
   c. thalassemia

   d. hemophilia
   e. none of the above

Answer:

28. Abnormal production of white blood cells is

    a. hemolytic
    b. leukemia
    c. thalassemia

    d. hemophilia
    e. none of the above

Answer:

29. Blood poisoning is

    a. septicemia
    b. malaria
    c. thalassemia

    d. anemia
    e. none of the above

Answer:

30. The Epstein-Barr virus causes

    a. septicemia
    b. malaria
    c. infectious mononucleosis

    d. sickle-cell anemia
    e. none of the above

Answer:

31. Carboxyhemoglobin forms when what substance binds to the iron atoms in hemoglobin?

    a. water
    b. oxygen
    c. carbon dioxide

    d. carbon monoxide
    e. nitrogen

Answer:

32. Which blood cells defend against allergens and worms?

    a. basophils
    b. neutrophils
    c. platelets

    d. erythrocytes
    e. eosinophils

Answer:

33. Iron-deficiency anemia can be caused by a deficiency of which vitamin?

    a. B12
    b. B6
    c. K

    d. E
    e. C

Answer:

CHAPTER 14

The Cardiovascular Circulatory System

OBJECTIVES

After studying this chapter, you should be able to:

1. Describe how the heart is positioned in the thoracic cavity.
2. List and describe the layers of the heart wall.
3. Name the chambers of the heart and their valves.
4. Name the major vessels that enter and exit the heart.
5. Describe blood flow through the heart.
6. Explain how the conduction system of the heart controls proper blood flow.
7. Describe the stages of a cardiac cycle.
8. Compare the anatomy of a vein, an artery, and a capillary.
9. Name the major blood circulatory routes.

ACTIVITIES

A. Completion

Fill in the blank spaces with the correct term.

1. The cardiovascular system consists of the ___ and the ___ ___.
2. ___ assist in the chemical reaction within cells.
3. Oxygen and nutrients from digested food help make the chemical energy ___.
4. Most of the heart is on the ___ side of the body's midline.

NAME: _____   DATE: _____

5. The membrane surrounding the heart is the ___ ___.

6. The outer layer of the membrane is the ___ ___, and the inferior inner layer is the ___ ___.

7. The outer layer of the heart is the ___.

8. The middle layer of the heart is the ___.

9. The inner layer of the heart is the ___.

10. The upper chambers of the heart are called the ___.

11. The lower chambers of the heart are called the ___.

12. The heart is separated into left and right sides by a(n) ___.

13. The three veins supplying blood to the right atrium are the ___ and ___ venae cavae and the ___ ___.

14. In the lungs, blood gives up ___ ___ and receives ___.

15. The heart muscle is supplied with blood by the ___.

16. The descending aorta becomes the ___ aorta.

17. Of the four heart chambers, the ___ ___ has the thickest walls.

18. There are ___ valves in the heart and these are the ___, ___, ___ ___, and the ___ ___.

19. All of the valves have three cusps except the ___, which has ___ cusps.

20. The superior vena cava drains the ___ portion of the body, and the inferior vena cava the ___ portion.

21. Deoxygenated blood is ___ ___ in color, whereas oxygenated blood is ___ ___.

22. The conduction system of the heart is actually a(n) ___ system.

23. The sinoatrial (SA) node is known as the ___.

24. The atrioventricular bundle is also known as the ___ of ___

25. The actual contractions of the ventricles are stimulated by ___ ___.

26. Regulation of the beats of the heart resides in the ___ ___ system.

27. Contraction of the heart is the ___, and the relaxation phase is the ___.

28. Blood supply to the heart is via the ___ ___ route.

29. The one temporary circulatory route is ___ ___.

30. The three layers of blood vessels are the ___, ___, and the ___.

31. ___ are small arteries.

32. ___ are small veins.

33. ___ are vessels consisting of a single cell layer.

34. The first branch of the aortic arch is the ___ artery.

35. The ___ arteries supply the head, neck, and brain.

36. A myocardial ___ results from the death of heart muscle cells caused by a blockage in coronary arteries.

37. After an angioplasty, a metal-mesh tube called a(n) ___ is inserted into the vessel.

38. ___ of the heart valves is a narrowed opening through the valves.

B. Matching

Match the term on the right with the definition on the left.

ARTERIES

_____ 39. divides into vertebral, axillary   a. celiac trunk and brachial arteries

_____ 40. 10 pairs   b. kidneys

_____ 41. supply the lungs   c. diaphragm

_____ 42. phrenic   d. bronchial

_____ 43. left gastric, splenic, common hepatic   e. internal iliac

_____ 44. right and left renal   f. intercostal

_____ 45. muscles of the abdomen   g. left subclavian

_____ 46. femoral, popliteal, tibial, dorsal pedis   h. lumbar

VEINS

_____ 47. drains the forearm   a. peroneal

_____ 48. connects to the axillary   b. azygos

_____ 49. where blood is drawn   c. hepatic

_____ 50. drains the thorax   d. radius and ulna

_____ 51. drains the calf and foot   e. external and internal iliac

_____ 52. merge with the femoral   f. cephalic

_____ 53. drains the pelvis   g. median cubital

_____ 54. drains the liver   h. saphenous

_____ 55. drains the digestive tract   i. hepatic portal

GENERAL

_____ 56. chest pain   a. heart failure

_____ 57. coronary thrombosis   b. congenital

_____ 58. does not pump enough blood   c. angina pectoris

_____ 59. heart disease present at birth   d. blood clot

C. Key Terms

Use the text to look up the following terms. Write the definition or explanation.

60. Abdominal aorta:

_____

_____

61. Anastomosis:

_____

_____

62. Anterior interventricular sulcus:

_____

_____

63. Aorta:

_____

_____

64. Aortic semilunar valve:

_____

_____

65. Arch of the aorta:

_____

_____

66. Arrhythmia:

_____

_____

67. Arteries:

_____

_____

68. Arterioles:

_____

_____

69. Ascending aorta:

_____

_____

70. Atherosclerosis:

_____

_____

71. Atrioventricular (AV) node:

_____

_____

72. Atrioventricular bundle/bundle of His:

_____

_____

73. Auricle:

_____

_____

74. Bicuspid/mitral valve:

_____

_____

75. Capillaries:

_____

_____

76. Cephalic vein:

_____

_____

77. Cerebral circulation:

_____

_____

78. Chordae tendineae:

_____

_____

79. Conduction myofibers:

_____

_____

80. Conduction system:

_____

_____

81. Coronary arteries:

_____

_____

82. Coronary circulation:

_____

_____

83. Coronary sinus:

_____

_____

84. Coronary sulcus:

_____

_____

85. Descending thoracic aorta:

_____

_____

86. Diastole:

_____

_____

87. Endocardium:

_____

_____

88. Epicardium:

_____

_____

89. Fetal circulation:

_____

_____

90. Fibrous pericardium:

_____

_____

91. Heart:

_____

_____

92. Hepatic portal circulation:

_____

_____

93. Inferior (posterior) vena cava:

_____

_____

94. Interventricular septum:

_____

_____

95. Left atrium:

_____

_____

96. Left bundle branch:

_____

_____

97. Left pulmonary artery:

_____

_____

98. Left ventricle:

_____

_____

99. Lumen:

_____

_____

100. Musculi pectinati:

_____

_____

101. Myocardium:

_____

_____

102. Pacemaker:

_____

_____

103. Papillary muscles:

_____

_____

104. Pericardial cavity:

_____

_____

105. Pericardial fluid:

_____

_____

106. Pericardial sac:

_____

_____

107. Posterior interventricular sulcus:

_____

_____

108. Pulmonary circulation:

_____

_____

109. Pulmonary semilunar valve:

_____

_____

110. Pulmonary trunk:

_____

_____

111. Pulmonary veins:

_____

_____

112. **P**urkinje's fibers/conduction myofibers:

_____

_____

113. **R**ight atrium:

_____

_____

114. **R**ight and left bundle branches:

_____

_____

115. **R**ight pulmonary artery:

_____

_____

116. **R**ight ventricle:

_____

_____

117. **S**erous pericardium:

_____

_____

118. **S**inoatrial (SA) node/pacemaker:

_____

_____

119. **S**uperior (anterior) vena cava:

_____

_____

120. **S**ystemic circulation:

_____

_____

121. **S**ystole:

_____

_____

122. Thoracic aorta:

_____

_____

123. Trabeculae carneae:

_____

_____

124. Tricuspid valve:

_____

_____

125. Tunica adventitia:

_____

_____

126. Tunica intima:

_____

_____

127. Tunica media:

_____

_____

128. Vascular:

_____

_____

129. Veins:

_____

_____

130. Venules:

_____

_____

D. Labeling Exercise

131. Label the chambers, vessels, valves, and septum of the heart as indicated in Figure 14-1.

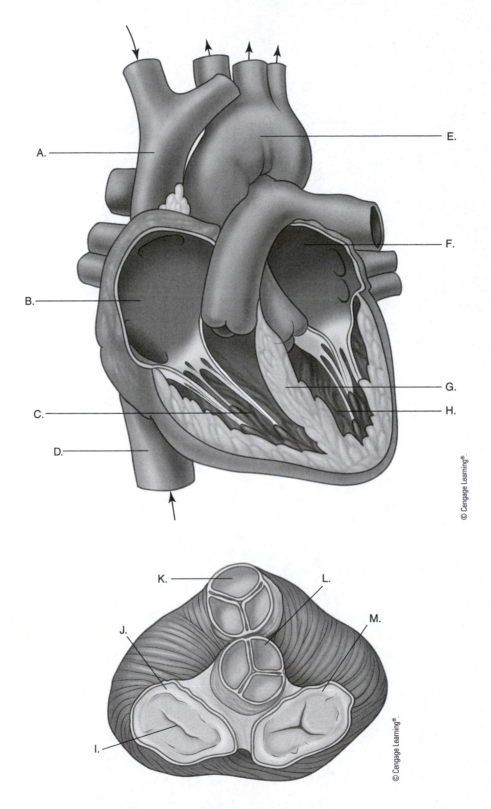

Figure 14-1

A. _____

B. _____

C. _____

D. _____

E. _____

F. _____

G. _____

H. _____

I. _____

J. _____

K. _____

L. _____

132. Label the arteries as indicated in Figure 14-2.

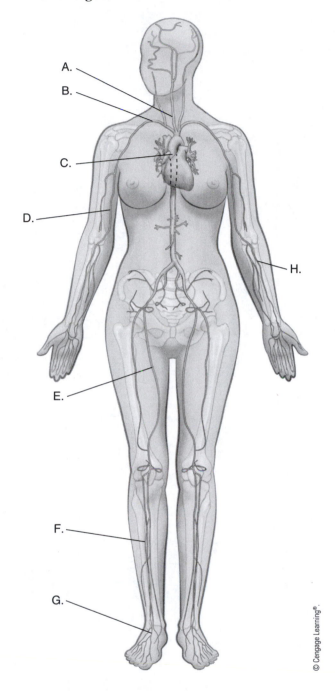

Figure 14-2

A. _____   E. _____

B. _____   F. _____

C. _____   G. _____

D. _____   H. _____

133. **Label the veins indicated in Figure 14-3.**

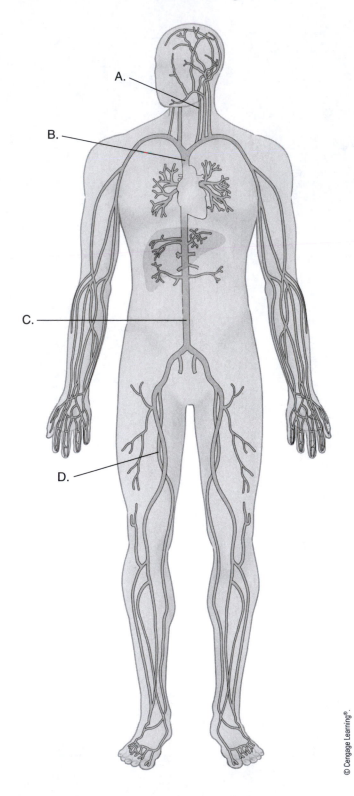

A. _____

B. _____

C. _____

D. _____

© Cengage Learning®.

Figure 14-3

E. Coloring Exercise

134. Using Figure 14-4, color the veins blue and the arteries red.

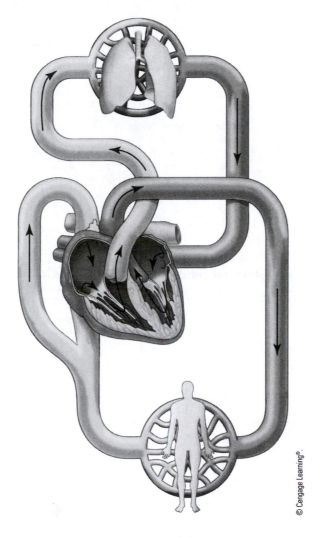

Figure 14-4

F. Critical Thinking

Answer the following questions in complete sentences.

135. Given a blood pressure reading of 130/86, which is the systole and which is the diastole?

136. If a person has angina pectoris and is probably having an MI, explain what may be happening to the heart.

137. Why is the saphenous vein used for heart bypass surgery?

138. How does the cardiovascular system integrate with the skin to control body temperature?

139. Why do our muscles tire during exercise?

140. How does the lymphatic system work with the cardiovascular system to protect the body?

141. Why does the blood not flow backward in our veins?

142. What does adrenaline do to our cardiovascular system?

143. How does the conduction system control proper blood flow?

144. Why does cardiac output of a 70-year-old person often decrease by 75%?

145. Why is walking one of the best exercises to maintain good heart performance?

146. Distinguish among a cardiovascular technologist, an electrocardiographic technician, and a cardiac sonographer.

G. Crossword Puzzle

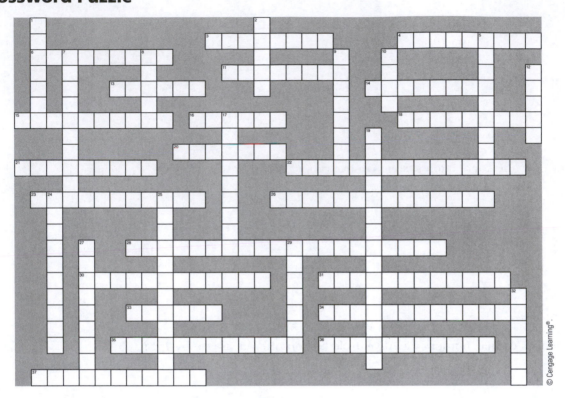

Complete the crossword puzzle using the following clues.

ACROSS

3. Another name for the mitral valve
4. SA node
6. 3-cusp valve regulating blood flow
11. Abnormal narrowing of the heart valve
13. Upper heart chamber
14. Relaxation phase of a heartbeat
15. Three veins that send blood to the right atrium
16. Carries oxygenated blood from the heart
18. Lower heart chamber
20. External appendage of the atrium
21. Smallest blood vessel
22. Supplies blood to the lungs
23. Thigh vein draining into the inferior vena cava
26. Subclavian artery
28. Heart attack
30. Inflammation of the pericardium

DOWN

1. Contraction phase of a heartbeat
2. Hollow core of a blood vessel
5. Small artery
7. Cardiac muscle layer
8. Largest artery
9. Hormone promoting female vascular health
10. Returns deoxygenated blood to the heart
12. Help protect CV organs
17. Valve between the right atrium and right ventricle
19. Arterial disease caused by plaque buildup
24. Outermost layer of heart
25. Inflammation of the inner heart layer
27. Longest vein
29. Area of damaged cardiac tissue
32. Small vein

31. High blood pressure

33. Organ supplied by the renal arteries

34. Helps maintain kidney function

35. Hole in the interatrial septum

36. Middle layer of the arterial wall

37. Junction of two or more blood vessels

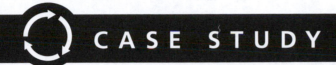
CASE STUDY

Ester, a 75-year-old woman, is admitted to an acute care facility with extreme shortness of breath and the feeling that she is suffocating. Upon preliminary assessment, the health care provider notes that Ester also has very swollen feet and ankles. When asked about her medical history, Ester states that she was diagnosed with high blood pressure around 8 years ago.

QUESTIONS

1. Based on her medical history and current symptoms, what condition might Ester have developed?

2. What pathological changes might be causing Ester's symptoms?

3. What are the major risk factors for the development of this disorder?

CHAPTER QUIZ

1. Which of the following is NOT transported by the blood?

   a. oxygen
   b. urine
   c. hormones
   d. waste
   e. nutrients

Answer:

2. The normal heartbeat is about how many times per minute?

   a. 60
   b. 100
   c. 90
   d. 72
   e. none of the above

Answer:

3. The heart is composed primarily of

    a. fat
    b. blood
    c. lymph

    d. muscle
    e. cartilage

Answer:

4. The serous pericardium is known as what layer of the pericardial sac?

    a. fibrous
    b. intima
    c. parietal

    d. visceral
    e. precordial

Answer:

5. The epicardium can also be referred to as the

    a. parietal pericardium
    b. pericardial cavity
    c. visceral peritoneum

    d. parietal peritoneum
    e. serous peritoneum

Answer:

6. The endocardium is made up of which type of tissue?

    a. epithelial
    b. connective
    c. muscle

    d. osseus
    e. none of the above

Answer:

7. The atrial appendage similar to a dog's ear is the

    a. auricle
    b. trabeculae
    c. septum

    d. bicuspid
    e. tricuspid

Answer:

8. The right atrium receives blood from all parts of the body EXCEPT the

    a. brain
    b. hands
    c. kidneys

    d. liver
    e. lungs

Answer:

9. The superior vena cava is also known as the

    a. small vena cava
    b. pulmonary vein
    c. posterior vena cava

    d. anterior vena cava
    e. coronary sinus

Answer:

10. The smallest of the four heart chambers is the

    a. right atrium
    b. left atrium
    c. right ventricle

    d. left ventricle
    e. coronary sinus

Answer:

11. The only heart valve with two cusps is the

a. tricuspid
b. mitral
c. pulmonary
d. aortic
e. semilunar

Answer:

12. Blood receives oxygen in the

a. liver
b. kidneys
c. lungs
d. heart
e. pancreas

Answer:

13. Blood deposits which of the following in the lungs?

a. oxygen
b. urine
c. hormones
d. carbon dioxide
e. renin

Answer:

14. Blood from the lungs returns to the heart through how many veins?

a. 2
b. 4
c. 6
d. 8
e. 3

Answer:

15. Blood from the lungs returns to which of the following?

a. right ventricle
b. left ventricle
c. right atrium
d. left atrium
e. superior vena cava

Answer:

16. An increase or a decrease in heart rate is controlled by which part of the nervous system?

a. central
b. autonomic
c. peripheral
d. forebrain
e. temporal

Answer:

17. Contraction of the ventricles is stimulated by the

a. SA node
b. AV node
c. bundle branches
d. bundle of His
e. Purkinje's fibers

Answer:

18. A cardiac cycle consists of contractions of

a. both atria
b. an atrium and a ventricle
c. two ventricles
d. two atria then two ventricles
e. all four chambers at once

Answer:

19. A complete cycle of blood flow is called

    a. pulmonary circulation
    b. coronary circulation
    c. hepatic portal circulation
    d. cerebral circulation
    e. systemic circulation

Answer:

20. Two major properties of arteries are

    a. irritability/contractility
    b. thickness/irritability
    c. hollowness/thinness
    d. elasticity/contractility
    e. anastomosis/fragility

Answer:

21. Which vessels have walls one cell thick?

    a. venules
    b. arteries
    c. capillaries
    d. arterioles
    e. veins

Answer:

22. Veins have something that arteries do not. Which of the following is it?

    a. irritability
    b. valves
    c. junctions
    d. smooth muscle
    e. contractility

Answer:

23. When the aorta arches and begins descending down along the spine, then goes through the diaphragm, it is known as the

    a. abdominal aorta
    b. thoracic aorta
    c. subclavian artery
    d. esophageal artery
    e. brachiocephalic artery

Answer:

24. The left common carotid artery branches from the

    a. right common carotid artery
    b. aortic arch
    c. left subclavian artery
    d. thoracic artery
    e. axillary artery

Answer:

25. The final branches of the abdominal aorta are the

    a. popliteal arteries
    b. femoral arteries
    c. common iliac arteries
    d. tibial arteries
    e. inferior mesenteric arteries

Answer:

26. Veins that drain the arm include all of the following EXCEPT the

    a. brachial
    b. cephalic
    c. vertebral
    d. basilic
    e. median cubital

Answer:

27. All of the following veins drain into the superior vena cava EXCEPT the

    a. internal jugular
    b. azygos
    c. internal iliac

    d. vertebral
    e. subclavian

Answer:

28. Which of the following does NOT drain into the inferior vena cava?

    a. azygos
    b. hepatic portal
    c. saphenous

    d. gonadal
    e. popliteal

Answer:

29. Which of the following is NOT an inflammatory condition?

    a. endocarditis
    b. atherosclerosis
    c. pericarditis

    d. gastritis
    e. myocarditis

Answer:

30. Two common congenital heart defects are

    a. thrombosis/angina
    b. hypertension/septal defect
    c. stenotic heart valves/hypertension

    d. angina/stenotic heart valves
    e. septal defect/stenotic heart valves

Answer:

31. From the AV node, a tract of conducting fibers runs through the cardiac mass to the top of the interventricular septum. This tract is called the

    a. bundle of His
    b. SA node
    c. right bundle branch

    d. conduction myofiber
    e. Purkinje's branch

Answer:

32. The major cause of death and heart disease in older Americans is

    a. heart arrythmia
    b. coronary artery disease
    c. an angioplasty

    d. a stenosed heart valve
    e. an incompetent heart valve

Answer:

33. What is the name for a slow heart beat rate of less than 60 beats per minute?

    a. angina
    b. hypertension
    c. bradycardia

    d. tachycardia
    e. septal defect

Answer:

The Lymphatic Circulatory System

OBJECTIVES

After studying this chapter, you should be able to:

1. Name the functions of the lymphatic system.
2. Explain what lymph is and how it forms.
3. Describe lymph flow through the body.
4. Name the principal lymphatic trunks.
5. Describe the functions of the tonsils and spleen.
6. Explain the unique role the thymus gland plays as part of the lymphatic system.
7. Describe the different types of immunity.
8. Explain the difference between blood and the lymphatic capillaries.
9. Explain the difference between active and passive immunity.
10. Define an *antigen* and an *antibody*.

ACTIVITIES

A. Completion

Fill in the blank spaces with the correct term.

1. The five organs of the lymphatic system are the ___, ___, ___, ___, and the ___ ___.
2. Interstitial fluid is ___ forced from capillaries.
3. Edema is another name for ___.
4. ___ is interstitial fluid that has entered a lymphatic capillary.
5. Chyle looks milky because of its ___ content.

NAME: _____   DATE: _____

6. The larger lymphatic vessels are the ___.

7. The larger lymphatic vessels of the viscera generally follow the routes of ___.

8. Efferent lymphatic vessels leave the lymph nodes at the ___.

9. Trabeculae are ___ ___.

10. Those vessels entering a lymph node are the ___ lymphatic vessels.

11. The lymph nodule surrounds a(n) ___ ___, which produces lymphocytes.

12. The stroma of a lymph node is made up of the ___, the ___, and the ___.

13. In the lymph node, any microorganisms or foreign substances stimulate ___ to divide, thereby activating the ___ ___.

14. Lymph trunks are formed by uniting ___ vessels.

15. The principal trunks pass their lymph into the ___ ___ and the ___ ___ ___.

16. The lymph flow cycle is completed when the lymph is drained back into the ___.

17. The ___ tonsils are the ones removed in a tonsillectomy.

18. The adenoids are the ___ tonsils.

19. The bilobed mass of tissue located in the mediastinum is the ___ ___.

20. In the spleen, ___ of worn-out red blood cells releases hemoglobin.

21. Peyer's patches are found in the wall of the ___ ___.

22. The ___ of the Peyer's patches destroy bacteria.

23. Disease-causing microorganisms are called ___

24. Plasma cells come from ___ ___.

25. High molecular weight proteins are the ___.

26. The body's production of antibodies against an antigen is ___ immunity.

27. The type of immunity received by the fetus from the mother is ___.

28. ___ ___ ___ destroy virus-invaded body cells.

29. ___ ___ is the disease of the lymphatic system with historical implications.

30. ___ is a tumor of the lymphatic system.

31. A vaccine contains either weak pathogens or ___ ___.

32. ___ engulf and digest antigens.

33. ___ ___ can be spread by growing in lymph nodes and being transported throughout the body by the lymphatic system.

B. Matching

Match the term on the right with the definition on the left.

_____ 34. lymph organs

_____ 35. interstitial fluid originally

_____ 36. lymphatic vessels in villi

_____ 37. chyle

a. lymphocytes

b. tonsillectomy

c. B lymphocytes

d. bubonic plague

_____ 38. aggregation of nodes   e. lymph trunk

_____ 39. capsular extension   f. Peyer's patches

_____ 40. lymph sinuses   g. milky lymph

_____ 41. germinal centers   h. plasma

_____ 42. efferent vessel union   i. tonsils

_____ 43. pharyngeal tonsils   j. trabeculae

_____ 44. palatine tonsils removed   k. lymphoma

_____ 45. aggregate lymph follicles   l. groin

_____ 46. provide humoral immunity   m. spaces

_____ 47. lymph tissue tumor   n. lacteals

_____ 48. *Klebsiella pestis*   o. adenoids

C. Key Terms

Use the text to look up the following terms. Write the definition or explanation.

49. Active immunity:

_____

_____

50. Afferent lymphatic vessels:

_____

_____

51. Allergies:

_____

_____

52. Antibodies/immunoglobulins:

_____

_____

53. Antigen:

_____

_____

54. B cells:

_____

_____

55. B lymphocytes:

_____

_____

56. Bone marrow transplants:

_____

_____

57. Bronchomediastinal trunk:

_____

_____

58. Cellular immunity:

_____

_____

59. Chyle:

_____

_____

60. Complement:

_____

_____

61. Cortical nodule/lymph nodule:

_____

_____

62. Edema:

_____

_____

63. Efferent lymphatic vessels:

_____

_____

64. Germinal center:

_____

_____

65. Helper T cells:

_____

_____

66. Hilum:

_____

_____

67. Humoral immunity:

_____

_____

68. Immunity:

_____

_____

69. Immunoglobulin A (IgA):

_____

_____

70. Immunoglobulin D (IgD):

_____

_____

71. Immunoglobulin E (IgE):

_____

_____

72. Immunoglobulin G (IgG):

_____

_____

73. Immunoglobulin M (IgM):

_____

_____

74. Intercostal trunk:

_____

_____

75. Interstitial fluid:

_____

_____

76. Intestinal trunk:

_____

_____

77. Jugular trunk:

_____

_____

78. Killer T cells:

_____

_____

79. Lacteals:

_____

_____

80. Lingual tonsils:

_____

_____

81. Lumbar trunk:

_____

_____

82. Lymph:

_____

_____

83. Lymphatic capillaries:

_____

_____

84. Lymph nodes/glands:

_____

_____

85. Lymphatic sinus:

_____

_____

86. Lymphatic trunks:

_____

_____

87. Lymphatics:

_____

_____

88. Lymphokines:

_____

_____

89. Lymphoma:

_____

_____

90. Macrophage:

_____

_____

91. Memory cells:

_____

_____

92. Monokines:

_____

_____

93. Palatine tonsils:

_____

_____

94. Passive immunity:

_____

_____

95. Pathogens:

_____

_____

96. Peyer's patches:

_____

_____

97. Pharyngeal tonsils/adenoids:

_____

_____

98. Plasma cells:

_____

_____

99. Right lymphatic duct:

_____

_____

100. Spleen:

_____

_____

101. Subclavian trunk:

_____

_____

102. Suppressor T cells:

_____

_____

103. Thoracic duct/left lymphatic duct:

_____

_____

104. Thymus gland:

_____

_____

105. T lymphocytes/T cells:

_____

_____

106. Trabeculae:

_____

_____

D. Labeling Exercise

107. Label the correct organs as indicated in Figure 15-1.

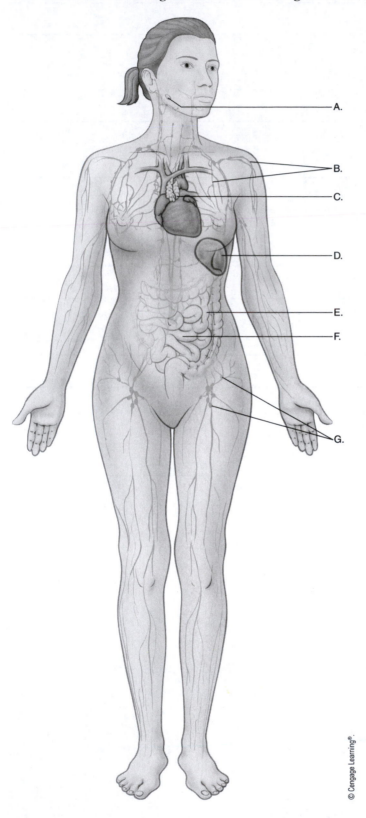

A.

B.

C.

D.

E.

F.

G.

A. _____

B. _____

C. _____

D. _____

E. _____

F. _____

G. _____

© Cengage Learning®.

Figure 15-1

108. Label the correct lymph nodes as indicated in Figure 15-2.

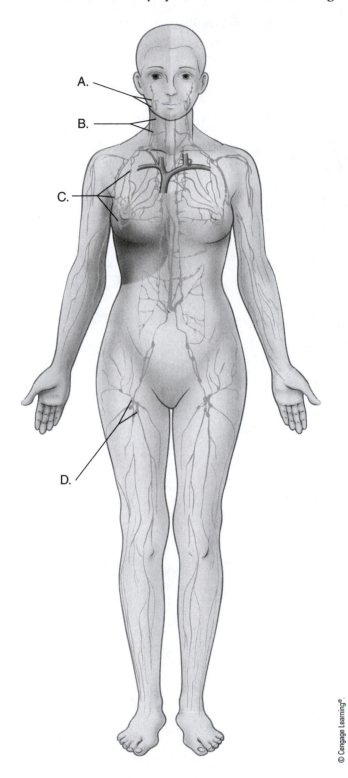

A. _____

B. _____

C. _____

D. _____

Figure 15-2

© Cengage Learning®

E. Coloring Exercise

109. Use Figure 15-3 to color the venule blue, the arteriole red, the blood capillary red, the lymphatic capillary green, and the interstitial fluid yellow.

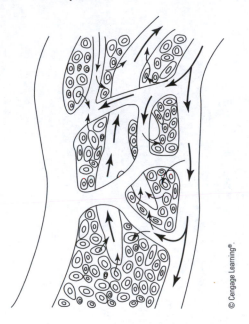

Figure 15-3

F. Critical Thinking

Answer the following questions in complete sentences.

110. Why can lymphatic vessels transport larger molecules than blood vessels?

111. Describe the framework of the lymph node.

112. Explain the immune response in a lymph node.

113. Differentiate elephantiasis in Africa and in Malaysia.

114. How does removal of the spleen affect immunity?

115. What are antibodies and how do they work?

116. Why does acquired immunodeficiency syndrome (AIDS) cause death by opportunistic diseases?

117. Explain the effect of age-related changes in the lymphatic system.

118. Differentiate between an immunologist and an oncologist.

G. Crossword Puzzle

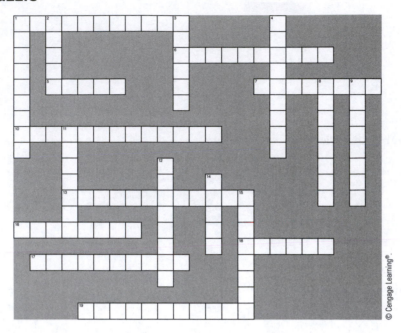

Complete the crossword puzzle using the following clues.

ACROSS

1. Engulf and digest antigens
5. Swelling
6. Large lymphatic vessels
7. Nodule of dense tissue in lymph node
10. Disease from blocked lymphatic system
13. Fluid found between tissue cells
16. Vessels entering lymph nodes
17. Enzymes that attack antigens
18. Formed by uniting efferent vessels
19. Chemical from T lymphocyte

DOWN

1. Chemicals released by macrophages
2. Lymph in lacteals
3. Single largest lymphatic tissue mass
4. Disease-causing microorganisms
8. Ability to resist infection
9. Pharyngeal tonsils
11. Immunity that is naturally conferred
12. Foreign proteins
14. Lymph node depression
15. Lymphatic vessels in intestinal villi

CASE STUDY

Mr. Delacruz, a 32-year-old man, is undergoing a routine physical examination. While examining his neck, the health care provider discovers enlarged lymph nodes that Mr. Delacruz reports are painless. He states that he noticed the enlarged nodes earlier, but ignored them because the nodes were not tender. The care provider makes an appointment for Mr. Delacruz with an oncologist for further evaluation.

QUESTIONS

1. What is the role of an oncologist?

2. What disorder might this patient have developed?

3. How is this condition usually treated?

4. What complications could Mr. Delacruz develop during the course of treatment?

CHAPTER QUIZ

1. Which cells are formed by replicating B cells?

   a. helper T cells
   b. plasma cells
   c. memory cells

   d. suppressor T cells
   e. none of the above

Answer:

2. Which cells exist in the body for years?

   a. helper T cells
   b. plasma cells
   c. memory cells

   d. suppressor T cells
   e. none of the above

Answer:

3. Which cells engulf and digest antigens?

   a. helper T cells
   b. plasma cells
   c. memory cells

   d. suppressor T cells
   e. none of the above

Answer:

4. Which cells bind with specific antigens presented by macrophages?

   a. helper T cells
   b. plasma cells
   c. memory cells

   d. suppressor T cells
   e. none of the above

Answer:

5. Inflammation of the lymphatic vessels is called

   a. lymphoma
   b. lymphadenitis
   c. lymphangitis

   d. bubonic plague
   e. none of the above

Answer:

6. The fluid that moves out of the blood capillaries is called

   a. lymph
   b. interstitial fluid
   c. plasma

   d. chyle
   e. none of the above

Answer:

7. When that fluid is in the lacteals, it is called

   a. lymph
   b. interstitial fluid
   c. plasma

   d. chyle
   e. none of the above

Answer:

8. Before the fluid leaves the blood capillaries, it is called

   a. lymph
   b. interstitial fluid
   c. plasma

   d. chyle
   e. none of the above

Answer:

9. The oval to bean-shaped structures of the lymphatic system are the

   a. lacteals
   b. vessels
   c. glands

   d. trabeculae
   e. none of the above

Answer:

10. The vessels entering a lymph node are the

    a. efferent
    b. trabeculae
    c. germinal

    d. afferent
    e. none of the above

Answer:

11. The structure producing lymphocytes and surrounded by the lymph nodule is the

    a. efferent
    b. trabeculae
    c. germinal

    d. afferent
    e. none of the above

Answer:

12. Which of the following helps make up the framework of the lymph node?

    a. efferent
    b. trabeculae
    c. germinal

    d. afferent
    e. none of the above

Answer:

13. The hilum is which of the following?

    a. efferent
    b. trabeculae
    c. germinal

    d. afferent
    e. none of the above

Answer:

14. The vessels that unite to form lymphatic trunks are the

    a. efferent
    b. trabeculae
    c. germinal

    d. afferent
    e. none of the above

Answer:

15. Which of the following is NOT one of the body's lymphatic trunks?

    a. lumbar
    b. thoracic
    c. bronchomediastinal

    d. subclavian
    e. jugular

Answer:

16. Which of the following drains lymph from the lower extremities?

    a. lumbar
    b. thoracic
    c. bronchomediastinal

    d. subclavian
    e. none of the above

Answer:

17. Which of the following is NOT a lymphatic trunk?

    a. thoracic
    b. jugular
    c. subclavian

    d. lumbar
    e. none of the above

Answer:

18. When the lymph cycle is complete, the fluid goes back to the

    a. nodes
    b. ducts
    c. lungs

    d. blood
    e. none of the above

Answer:

19. Which of the following are NOT tonsils?

    a. palatine
    b. adenoids
    c. lingual

    d. pharyngeal
    e. none of the above

Answer:

20. Which of the following is NOT a lymph organ?

    a. tonsils
    b. spleen
    c. thymus

    d. Peyer's patches
    e. none of the above

Answer:

21. The aggregated lymphatic follicles are the

    a. tonsils
    b. spleen
    c. thymus

    d. Peyer's patches
    e. none of the above

Answer:

22. Immunity produced by the body's lymphoid tissue is

    a. passive
    b. inherited
    c. cellular

    d. injected
    e. none of the above

Answer:

23. Which of the following gamma globulins activates complement?

    a. G
    b. A
    c. M

    d. D
    e. none of the above

Answer:

24. Which of the following gamma globulins is important in B-cell activation?

    a. G
    b. A
    c. M

    d. D
    e. none of the above

Answer:

25. Which of the following gamma globulins develops in blood plasma?

    a. G
    b. A
    c. M

    d. D
    e. none of the above

Answer:

26. Interleukin-1 stimulates T cell proliferation and causes fever. It is a(n)

    a. lymphokine
    b. monokine
    c. immunoglobulin

    d. interferon
    e. none of the above

Answer:

27. The thymus gland decreases in size as we age. It is replaced with

    a. muscle tissue
    b. adipose tissue
    c. nervous tissue

    d. tendons
    e. bone

Answer:

28. Eight times as many women than men develop

    a. SLE
    b. cancer
    c. allergies

    d. lymphadenitis
    e. lymphangitis

Answer:

Nutrition and the Digestive System

OBJECTIVES

After studying this chapter, you should be able to:

1. List and describe the five basic activities of the digestive process.

2. List the four layers or tunics of the walls of the digestive tract.

3. Name the major and accessory organs of the digestive tract and their component anatomic parts.

4. Explain the major digestive enzymes and how they function.

5. Explain the functions of the liver.

6. Explain how absorption of nutrients occurs in the small intestine and how the feces form in the large intestine.

7. Name and describe the functions of the organs of the digestive tract.

ACTIVITIES

A. Completion

Fill in the blank spaces with the correct term.

1. Breaking down food into simpler substances that the cells can use is the process of ___.

2. Mastication is the process of ___.

3. ___ plus lipase plus water produces glycerol.

4. The digestion of food begins in the mouth through the action of the enzyme ___.

5. The lining of the entire alimentary canal has ___ layers or ___.

NAME: _____   DATE: _____

6. The tunica muscularis is responsible for propelling food along by ___.

7. The mesentery is an extension of the ___ ___.

8. The anterior part of the roof of the mouth is the ___ ___.

9. The lingual frenulum is a(n) ___ dividing the tongue.

10. The tongue is supported by the ___ bone.

11. Saliva is mostly water, but an important chemical activator in it is ___.

12. If the mumps virus infects the pancreas, it can cause ___.

13. The ___ extend slightly into each tooth socket.

14. Infants' teeth are called ___ teeth.

15. Teeth can have as many as ___ root projections.

16. Tooth decay is also called ___ ___.

17. There are three parts to the pharynx; they are the ___, ___, and the ___.

18. The tube connecting the laryngopharynx and the stomach is the ___, which passes through the ___ and ___.

19. The stomach begins with the ___ and ends at the ___.

20. The small intestine begins with the ___ and ends with the ___.

21. An ulcer can be caused by either excess ___ or ___.

22. Alpha and beta cells of the pancreas secrete ___ and ___.

23. Another cell of the pancreas secretes enzymes; this is the ___.

24. There are ___ major functions of the liver.

25. The functions of the gallbladder are ___ and ___.

26. The walls of the small intestine are protected from digestion by ___.

27. The folds of the small intestine are called ___, and the projections are called ___.

28. The bowel begins with the ___ and ends at the ___ canal.

29. The end of the alimentary canal is the ___.

30. The final act of the digestive system is ___.

31. Hepatitis can be caused by virus ___ or virus ___.

32. Gallstones are caused by ___.

33. A chronic, inflammatory bowel disease with unknown origin is ___ ___.

34. Diverticulosis is a disorder characterized by ___ in the muscular layer of the colon.

35. Inflammation and enlargement of rectal veins is ___ or ___.

36. The taste of ___ was identified by Japanese researchers. It detects the flavor of MSG.

37. Stomach cancer produces gastric tumors called ___.

38. ___ cancer is an uncommon but deadly cancer. It occurs more often in men than in women.

B. Matching

Match the term on the right with the definition on the left.

_____ 39. degenerative liver disease

_____ 40. inflammatory bowel disease

_____ 41. rectal vein enlargement

_____ 42. digested food to the cardiovascular system

_____ 43. gastrointestinal tract

_____ 44. visceral peritoneum

_____ 45. posterior roof of the mouth

_____ 46. septum divides the tongue

_____ 47. important in licking

_____ 48. salivary enzyme

_____ 49. premolar

_____ 50. three cusps

_____ 51. enamel covered

_____ 52. tube behind the trachea

_____ 53. rounded portion above the cardia

_____ 54. principal gastric enzyme

_____ 55. duct of Wirsung

_____ 56. second portion of the large intestine

_____ 57. first part of the large intestine

_____ 58. colon joins the rectum

a. lingual frenulum

b. sigmoid colon

c. bicuspids

d. amylase

e. filiform papillae

f. cecum

g. pepsinogen

h. fundus

i. jejunum

j. pancreatic duct

k. soft palate

l. Crohn's disease

m. absorption

n. esophagus

o. hemorrhoids

p. cirrhosis

q. tricuspid

r. tunica serosa

s. crown

t. alimentary canal

C. Key Terms

Use the text to look up the following terms. Write the definition or explanation.

59. Absorption:

_____

_____

60. Acini:

_____

_____

61. Adventitia:

_____

_____

62. Alimentary canal:

_____

_____

63. Ampulla of Vater/hepatopancreatic ampulla:

_____

_____

64. Amylase:

_____

_____

65. Anal canal:

_____

_____

66. Anal columns:

_____

_____

67. Anus:

_____

_____

68. Apical foramen:

_____

_____

69. Ascending colon:

_____

_____

70. Bicuspids:

_____

_____

71. Bile duct:

_____

_____

72. Bowel:

_____

_____

73. Brunner's glands/duodenal glands:

_____

_____

74. Buccal glands:

_____

_____

75. Canine teeth:

_____

_____

76. Cardia:

_____

_____

77. Cecum:

_____

_____

78. Cementum:

_____

_____

79. Cervix/neck:

_____

_____

80. Chyme:

_____

_____

81. Circumvallate papillae:

_____

_____

82. Colon:

_____

_____

83. Crown:

_____

_____

84. Crypt of Lieberkuhn:

_____

_____

85. Cuspids:

_____

_____

86. Defecation:

_____

_____

87. Deglutition:

_____

_____

88. Dentes:

_____

_____

89. Dentin:

_____

_____

90. Descending colon:

_____

_____

91. Diaphragm:

_____

_____

92. Diarrhea:

_____

_____

93. Digestion:

_____

_____

94. Duct of Wirsung/pancreatic duct:

_____

_____

95. Duodenum:

_____

_____

96. Enamel:

_____

_____

97. *Entamoeba histolytica*:

_____

_____

98. *Escherichia coli*:

_____

_____

99. Esophageal hiatus:

_____

_____

100. Esophagus:

_____

_____

101. Falciform ligament:

_____

_____

102. Feces:

_____

_____

103. Filiform papillae:

_____

_____

104. Food bolus:

_____

_____

105. Fundus:

_____

_____

106. Fungiform papillae:

_____

_____

107. Gallbladder:

_____

_____

108. Gastroesophageal sphincter:

_____

_____

109. Gastrointestinal tract:

_____

_____

110. Gingivae:

_____

_____

111. Glucagon:

_____

_____

112. Glycogen:

_____

_____

113. Hard palate:

_____

_____

114. Haustrae:

_____

_____

115. *Helicobacter pylori*:

_____

_____

116. Heparin:

_____

_____

117. Ileocecal valve:

_____

_____

118. Ileum:

_____

_____

119. Incisors:

_____

_____

120. Ingestion:

_____

_____

121. Insulin:

_____

_____

122. Intestinal glands:

_____

_____

123. Islets of Langerhans/pancreatic islets:

_____

_____

124. Jejunum:

_____

_____

125. Kupffer's cells:

_____

_____

126. Lamina propria:

_____

_____

127. Large intestine/bowel:

_____

_____

128. Left colic (splenic) flexure:

_____

_____

129. Lingual frenulum:

_____

_____

130. Lips:

_____

_____

131. Liver:

_____

_____

132. Lower esophageal sphincter:

_____

_____

133. Mastication:

_____

_____

134. Mediastinum:

_____

_____

135. Mesentery:

_____

_____

136. Mesocolon:

_____

_____

137. Microvilli:

_____

_____

138. Molar teeth:

_____

_____

139. Mucous cells:

_____

_____

140. Mumps:

_____

_____

141. Muscularis mucosa:

_____

_____

142. Nasopharynx:

_____

_____

143. Oropharynx:

_____

_____

144. Pancreas:

_____

_____

145. Pancreatic juice:

_____

_____

146. Papillae:

_____

_____

147. Parietal cells:

_____

_____

148. Parotid gland:

_____

_____

149. Pepsin:

_____

_____

150. Pepsinogen:

_____

_____

151. Periodontal ligament:

_____

_____

152. Peristalsis:

_____

_____

153. Pharynx:

_____

_____

154. Plicae:

_____

_____

155. Premolars:

_____

_____

156. Prothrombin:

_____

_____

157. Pulp cavity:

_____

_____

158. Pyloric sphincter:

_____

_____

159. Pylorus/antrum:

_____

_____

160. Rectum:

_____

_____

161. Right colic (hepatic) flexure:

_____

_____

162. Root:

_____

_____

163. Root canals:

_____

_____

164. Rugae:

_____

_____

165. Sigmoid colon:

_____

_____

166. Small intestine:

_____

_____

167. Soft palate:

_____

_____

168. Sublingual gland:

_____

_____

169. Submandibular/submaxillary gland:

_____

_____

170. Submucosa:

_____

_____

171. Thrombin:

_____

_____

172. Tongue:

_____

_____

173. Transverse colon:

_____

_____

174. Tricuspids:

_____

_____

175. Tunica mucosa:

_____

_____

176. Tunica muscularis:

_____

_____

177. Tunica serosa:

_____

_____

178. Tunica submucosa:

_____

_____

179. Uvula:

_____

_____

180. Vermiform appendix:

_____

_____

181. Villi:

_____

_____

182. Visceral peritoneum:

_____

_____

183. Zymogenic/chief cells:

_____

_____

D. Labeling Exercise

184. Label the parts of the digestive system as indicated in Figure 16-1.

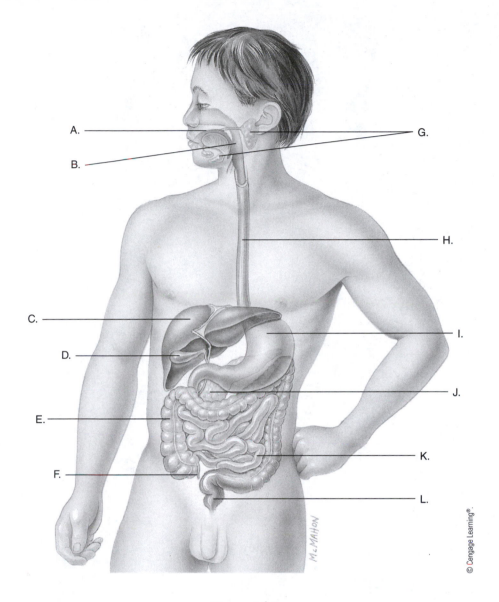

Figure 16-1

A. _____

B. _____

C. _____

D. _____

E. _____

F. _____

G. _____

H. _____

I. _____

J. _____

K. _____

L. _____

185. Label the parts of the stomach and the small intestine as indicated in Figure 16-2.

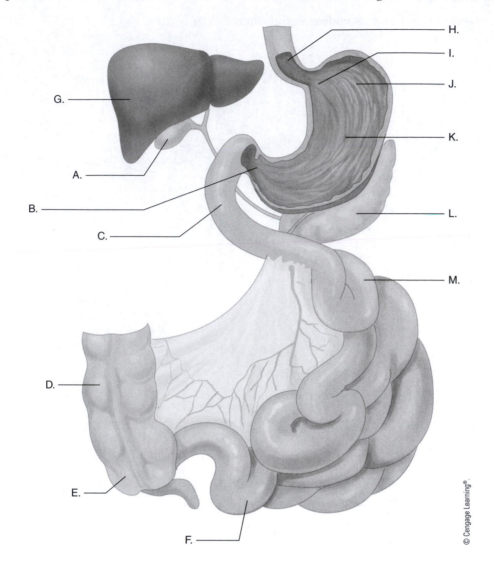

Figure 16-2

A. _____   H. _____

B. _____   I. _____

C. _____   J. _____

D. _____   K. _____

E. _____   L. _____

F. _____   M. _____

G. _____

E. Coloring Exercise

186. Using Figure 16-3, color the ascending colon red, the transverse colon green, the descending colon yellow, the sigmoid colon brown, the rectum orange, and the cecum blue.

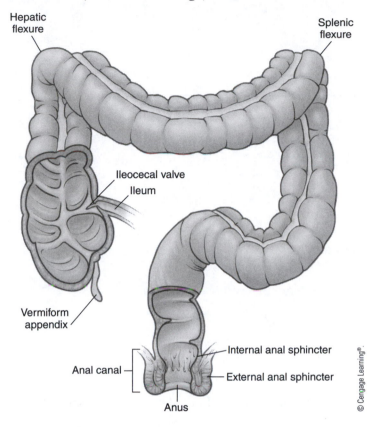

Figure 16-3

F. Critical Thinking

Answer the following questions in complete sentences.

187. Why do cavities occur?

188. Explain the first stage of digestion.

189. Why does food stuck in the esophagus cause breathing difficulties?

190. Why does a hiatal hernia cause a burning sensation in the esophagus?

191. Explain the formation of an ulcer.

192. Incomplete development of the hard palate (cleft palate) causes nasality. Why?

193. How does the pancreas contribute to the digestive process?

194. Explain absorption in the small intestine.

195. As people age, why do they become more susceptible to digestive system disorders?

196. Of the career opportunities presented, choose one that is the most interesting to you. Explain why.

G. True or False

Write "True" or "False" on the line provided.

197. _____ Vitamin E is necessary for the mineralization of bone tissue.

198. _____ Thiamine is another name for vitamin B_1.

H. Crossword Puzzle

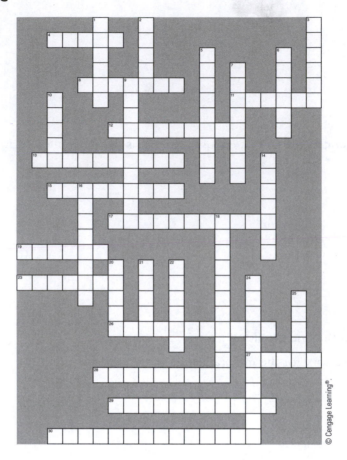

Complete the crossword puzzle using the following clues.

ACROSS

4. One of the largest organs of the digestive system
8. Anticoagulant
11. Tooth that tears food
12. Inflammation of the liver
13. Waste elimination
15. Breakdown of food
17. Stores bile
19. Teeth are made of it
23. Breaks down starch in the mouth
26. Chewing
27. Stomach folds
28. Taking in food
29. Pushing food along
30. Pouchlike herniation

DOWN

1. Teeth
2. Tooth that grinds food
3. Folds of the intestine
5. Extension of the visceral peritoneum
6. 99.5% H_2O
7. Teeth that cut food
9. Tunica serosa
10. Semifluid in the intestine
14. Connects with the duodenum
16. Gums
18. Swallowing
20. First part of large intestine
21. Disease of the salivary glands
22. Between the crown and root
24. Enlarged rectal veins
25. Hangs from the palate

Chapter 16 • *Nutrition and the Digestive System*   **341**

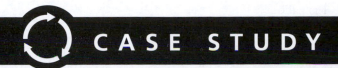

CASE STUDY

Bill Martin, a 19-year-old male student, is brought into the emergency room by his college roommates. Bill tells the health care provider that he started developing lower right abdominal pain while playing basketball. He states that his pain is becoming more severe. Based on his symptoms and the results of diagnostic studies, Bill is scheduled for emergency abdominal surgery.

QUESTIONS

1. Why is Bill experiencing severe lower right abdominal pain?

2. Where is the structure located that is causing Bill's symptoms?

3. Why is this structure prone to the development of obstruction and other problems?

4. Why must Bill undergo emergency abdominal surgery?

CHAPTER QUIZ

1. An inflammation of the liver that can be caused by alcohol or a virus is called

   a. cirrhosis
   b. Crohn's disease
   c. hepatitis

   d. diverticulosis
   e. none of the above

Answer:

2. When the liver becomes scarred and degenerates, it is called

   a. cirrhosis
   b. Crohn's disease
   c. hepatitis

   d. diverticulosis
   e. none of the above

Answer:

3. A chronic, inflammatory bowel disease is called

   a. cirrhosis
   b. Crohn's disease
   c. hepatitis

   d. diverticulosis
   e. none of the above

Answer:

© 2016 Cengage Learning. All Rights Reserved. May not be scanned, copied or duplicated, or posted to a publicly accessible website, in whole or in part.

4. When the bowel has pouchlike herniations, it is called

   a. cirrhosis
   b. Crohn's disease
   c. hepatitis

   d. diverticulosis
   e. none of the above

Answer:

5. The movement of food through the alimentary canal by smooth muscles is called

   a. ingestion
   b. digestion
   c. mastication

   d. peristalsis
   e. none of the above

Answer:

6. Taking food into the body is called

   a. ingestion
   b. digestion
   c. mastication

   d. peristalsis
   e. none of the above

Answer:

7. The act of swallowing is called

   a. deglutition
   b. mastication
   c. ingestion

   d. peristalsis
   e. none of the above

Answer:

8. Which of the following is NOT an accessory structure of the gastrointestinal tract?

   a. teeth
   b. tongue
   c. liver

   d. salivary glands
   e. none of the above

Answer:

9. Which of the following is NOT one of the four tunics of the alimentary canal?

   a. tunica mucosa
   b. lamina propria
   c. muscularis

   d. serosa
   e. none of the above

Answer:

10. Which of the papillae are important in licking?

    a. fungiform
    b. circumvallate
    c. filiform

    d. frenulum
    e. none of the above

Answer:

11. The salivary glands that secrete the least amount of saliva are the

    a. parotids
    b. submandibular
    c. buccal

    d. sublingual
    e. none of the above

Answer:

12. Which of the following substances is NOT found in saliva?

    a. amylase
    b. urea
    c. lipase

    d. phosphates
    e. none of the above

Answer:

13. The number of permanent teeth is

    a. 20
    b. 13
    c. 24

    d. 32
    e. none of the above

Answer:

14. Cavities are known as

    a. dentes
    b. gingivae
    c. pulp

    d. caries
    e. none of the above

Answer:

15. Which of the following are NOT teeth?

    a. molar
    b. canine
    c. incisor

    d. cuspid
    e. none of the above

Answer:

16. All of the following are parts of the pharynx EXCEPT

    a. tracheo
    b. naso
    c. oro

    c. laryngo
    e. none of the above

Answer:

17. The major symptom of a hiatal hernia is

    a. tickling
    b. raspiness
    c. burning

    d. pressure
    e. none of the above

Answer:

18. All of the following are parts of the stomach EXCEPT

    a. cardia
    b. fundus
    c. pylorus

    d. antrum
    e. none of the above

Answer:

19. All of the following are secretion cells of the stomach EXCEPT

    a. zymogenic
    b. alpha
    c. parietal

    d. mucous
    e. none of the above

Answer:

20. The folds of the stomach are called

    a. pepsin
    b. HCl
    c. rugae

    d. pepsinogen
    e. none of the above

Answer:

21. Approximately 80% of nutrient absorption takes place in the

    a. stomach
    b. small intestine
    c. large intestine

    d. liver
    e. none of the above

Answer:

22. Digestion of protein begins in the

    a. stomach
    b. pancreas
    c. liver

    d. large intestine
    e. none of the above

Answer:

23. Which of the following is NOT a function of the liver?

    a. produces heparin
    b. phagocytoses blood cells
    c. stores excess carbohydrates

    d. produces bile salts
    e. absorbs water

Answer:

24. All of the following are parts of the small intestine EXCEPT

    a. duodenum
    b. cecum
    c. jejunum

    d. ileum
    e. plicae

Answer:

25. The absorption structures of the small intestine are

    a. villi
    b. plicae
    c. chyme

    d. rugae
    e. none of the above

Answer:

26. The valves of the alimentary canal are of which type?

    a. flap
    b. cusp
    c. bicusp

    d. sphincter
    e. none of the above

Answer:

27. Which large intestinal movement mixes the chyme and helps in the absorption of water?

    a. peristalsis
    b. mass peristalsis
    c. vibration

    d. haustral churning
    e. none of the above

Answer:

28. Which of the following is NOT a part of the colon?

    a. rectum
    b. ascending
    c. sigmoid

    d. transverse
    e. descending

Answer:

29. Which of the following is NOT a function of the large intestine?

    a. water absorption
    b. feces formation
    c. vitamin production

    d. mucus production
    e. digestive enzyme secretion

Answer:

30. Which of the following is the end of the alimentary canal?

    a. sigmoid
    b. rectum
    c. anus

    d. descending colon
    e. none of the above

Answer:

31. Which of the following is a pear-shaped sac located in a depression of the liver surface?

    a. gallbladder
    b. colon
    c. parotid gland

    d. villi
    e. jejunum

Answer:

32. Which of the following is an indication of stomach ulcers or cancer?

    a. GERD
    b. tapeworm infection
    c. jaundice

    d. chronic gastritis
    e. chronic pancreatitis

Answer:

33. GERD causes a burning sensation in the esophagus because gastric juice is high in

    a. sugars
    b. water
    c. ammonia

    d. sulfuric acid
    e. hydrochloric acid

Answer:

The Respiratory System

OBJECTIVES

After studying this chapter, you should be able to:

1. Explain the function of the respiratory system.

2. Name the organs of the system.

3. Define the parts of the internal nose and their functions.

4. Name the three areas of the pharynx and explain their anatomy.

5. Name the cartilages and membranes of the larynx and how they function.

6. Explain how the anatomy of the trachea prevents collapse during breathing and allows for esophageal expansion during swallowing.

7. Explain what is meant by the term *bronchial tree*.

8. Describe the structure and function of the lungs and pleura.

9. Describe the overall process of gas exchange in the lungs and tissues.

10. Define ventilation, external respiration, and internal respiration.

ACTIVITIES

A. Completion

Fill in the blank spaces with the correct term.

1. There are two systems responsible for supplying oxygen and eliminating carbon dioxide; they are the ___ and the ___ systems.

2. The bridge of the nose is formed by the ___ bones.

NAME: _____   DATE: _____

3. The underside of the external nose has two openings called ___.

4. Posteriorly, the internal nose connects with the ___.

5. The nasal septum divides the left and right ___ ___.

6. The interior structures of the nose have ___ functions.

7. Olfactory receptors are located in the membrane of the ___ meatus.

8. The adenoid tonsils are located in the posterior wall of the ___ ___.

9. The opening of the oropharynx is called the ___.

10. The voice box is the ___.

11. The epiglottis forms a lid over the ___.

12. The paired rod-shaped cartilage structures of the larynx are the ___ cartilages.

13. The false vocal cords are the ___ ___.

14. The goblet cells of the trachea produce ___.

15. There are 16 to 20 incomplete rings of ___ cartilage in the trachea.

16. The lobar bronchi are the ___ bronchi, and the segmental bronchi are the ___ bronchi.

17. The pleural membrane covering the wall of the cavity is the ___, and the membrane covering the lungs is the ___.

18. The air sacs where gas exchange takes place are the ___.

19. Movement of air between the atmosphere and the lungs is called ___.

20. Internal respiration is the exchange of gases between the blood and ___.

21. ___ ___ affects the secretory cells of the lungs.

22. Any infection in the lungs is known as ___.

23. Whooping cough is also known as ___.

24. The disease caused by excessive exposure to asbestos, silica, or coal dust is ___ ___.

25. Bronchitis causes a swelling of the ___ ___ of the bronchi.

26. Respiratory distress syndrome is also known as ___ ___ disease.

27. Laryngitis is an inflammation of the mucosal membrane lining of the ___.

28. ___ can result from a loss of pressure in the lung or reduced elastic recoil of a lung.

B. Matching

Match the term on the right with the definition on the left.

___ 29. food convert to ATP   a. epiglottis

___ 30. internal nose to pharynx   b. oropharynx

___ 31. separates nasal cavities   c. cystic fibrosis

___ 32. sense of smell   d. thyroid cartilage

___ 33. another name for auditory tubes   e. vocal folds

___ 34. passage for food and air   f. pleural membrane

___ 35. single piece in the larynx   g. tertiary bronchi

_____ 36. Adam's apple

_____ 37. leaf-shaped cartilage

_____ 38. paired, cone-shaped

_____ 39. false vocal cords

_____ 40. true vocal cords

_____ 41. primary bronchi divide into

_____ 42. segmented bronchi

_____ 43. enclose and protect the lungs

_____ 44. space between the membranes

_____ 45. gases diffuse through it

_____ 46. exchange gas between blood cells

_____ 47. cavities inside the nostrils

_____ 48. affects the secretion cells of the lungs

h. corniculate cartilage

i. internal respiration

j. cricoid cartilage

k. nasal septum

l. lobar bronchi

m. olfactory stimuli

n. respiratory membrane

o. eustachian tubes

p. cellular respiration

q. internal nares

r. pleural cavity

s. vestibules

t. vestibular folds

C. Key Terms

Use the text to look up the following terms. Write the definition or explanation.

49. Alveolar-capillary membrane/respiratory membrane:

_____

_____

50. Alveolar ducts/atria:

_____

_____

51. Alveolar sacs:

_____

_____

52. Alveoli:

_____

_____

53. Arytenoid cartilages:

_____

_____

54. Auditory/eustachian tube:

_____

_____

55. Bronchial tree:

_____

_____

56. Bronchioles:

_____

_____

57. Bronchopulmonary segment:

_____

_____

58. Corniculate cartilage:

_____

_____

59. Cricoid cartilage:

_____

_____

60. Cuneiform cartilage:

_____

_____

61. Emphysema:

_____

_____

62. Epiglottis:

_____

_____

63. Exhalation/expiration:

_____

_____

64. External respiration:

_____

_____

65. Fauces:

_____

_____

66. Glottis:

_____

_____

67. Inferior meatus:

_____

_____

68. Inhalation/inspiration:

_____

_____

69. Internal nares:

_____

_____

70. Internal respiration:

_____

_____

71. Laryngopharynx:

_____

_____

72. Larynx:

_____

_____

73. Left primary bronchus:

_____

_____

74. Lobules:

_____

_____

75. Middle meatus:

_____

_____

76. Nasal cavities:

_____

_____

77. Nasal septum:

_____

_____

78. Nasopharynx:

_____

_____

79. Nostrils/external nares:

_____

_____

80. Olfactory stimuli:

_____

_____

81. Oropharynx:

_____

_____

82. Parietal pleura:

_____

_____

83. Partial pressure:

_____

_____

84. Pharynx:

_____

_____

85. Pleural cavity:

_____

_____

86. Pleural membrane:

_____

_____

87. Pleurisy/pleuritis:

_____

_____

88. Respiration:

_____

_____

89. Respiratory bronchioles:

_____

_____

90. Right primary bronchus:

_____

_____

91. Secondary/lobar bronchi:

_____

_____

92. Superior meatus:

_____

_____

93. Surfactant:

_____

_____

94. Terminal bronchioles:

_____

_____

95. Tertiary/segmental bronchi:

_____

_____

96. Thyroid cartilage/Adam's apple:

_____

_____

97. Trachea:

_____

_____

98. Ventilation/breathing:

_____

_____

99. Vestibular folds/false vocal cords:

_____

_____

100. Vestibules:

_____

_____

101. Visceral pleura:

_____

_____

102. Vocal folds/true vocal cords:

_____

_____

D. Labeling Exercise

103. Label the parts of the respiratory system as indicated in Figure 17-1.

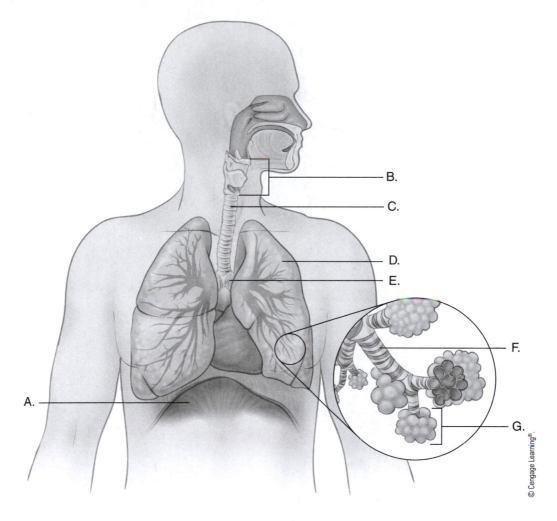

Figure 17-1

A. _____ F. _____

B. _____ G. _____

C. _____ H. _____

D. _____ I. _____

E. _____

104. Label the parts of the nasal cavity and pharynx as indicated in Figure 17-2.

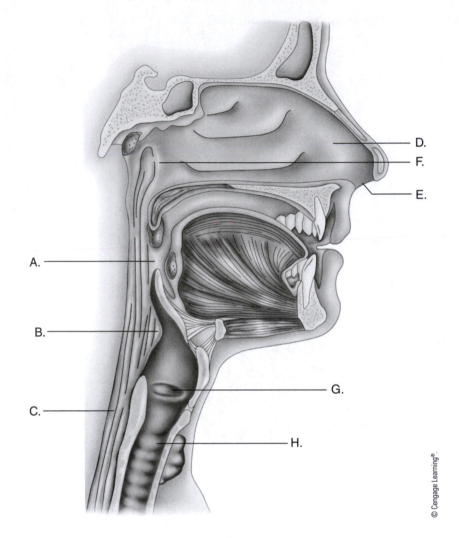

Figure 17-2

A. _____

B. _____

C. _____

D. _____

E. _____

F. _____

G. _____

H. _____

E. Coloring Exercise

105. Using Figure 17-3, color the thyroid cartilage green, the lungs blue, and the primary bronchus orange.

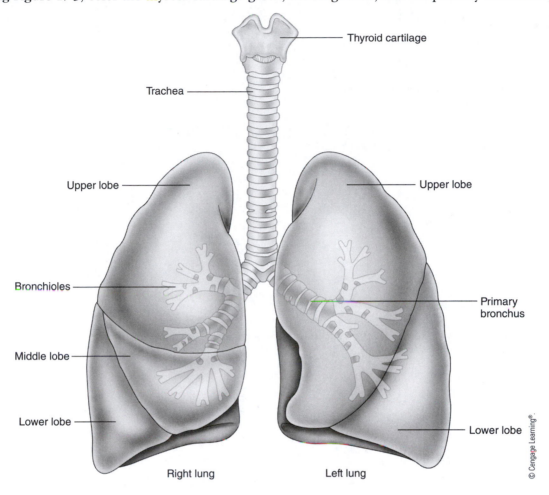

Figure 17-3

F. Critical Thinking

Answer the following questions in complete sentences.

106. How is the nose the first line of defense against foreign material?

107. How does material inadvertently enter the trachea?

108. What are the functions of the C rings of cartilage in the trachea?

109. Why is it called the "bronchial tree"?

110. Explain emphysema.

111. How do the nervous system and the respiratory system assist each other?

112. Explain fetal respiration.

113. What effect will age-related changes have on the respiratory system?

114. Using an online reference, identify the types of activities performed by a respiratory therapist.

G. Crossword puzzle

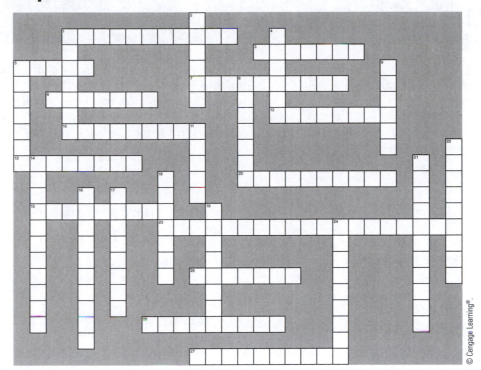

Complete the crossword puzzle using the following clues.

ACROSS

  1. Cone-shaped cartilage

  3. Adam's apple cartilage

  5. Alveolar ducts

  6. Many small compartments

  7. Covers glottis

10. Breathing muscle

12. Segmented bronchi

13. Carries oxygen

15. Lung infection

20. Prevents collapse of alveoli

23. Converts food to ATP

25. Tubes from the trachea to the lungs

26. Destruction of alveoli walls

27. Anterior nasal cavities

DOWN

  1. Cartilage of larynx

  2. Opening of oropharynx

  4. Pharynx

  5. Air sacs

  8. Space between vocal cords

  9. Voice box

11. Shelf passageways

14. Exchange of gases

16. Nasal cavity bones

17. External nares

18. Windpipe

19. Pleuritis

21. Breathing

22. Ladle-shaped cartilage

24. Whooping cough

CASE STUDY

During a smog alert, Liam, a 60-year-old man, is admitted to the emergency room. Liam, who was walking around outdoors during the alert, is experiencing extreme shortness of breath. Physical assessment reveals that Liam has an enlarged thoracic cavity. Liam states he has been smoking at least two packs of cigarettes a day since adolescence. He also says that he has been trying various smoking cessation programs for years without success. Liam is transferred to the medical unit and the admitting nurse notifies Liam's pulmonologist about his condition.

QUESTIONS

1. Given his symptoms and history, what condition do you think Liam might have developed?

2. What are the major risk factors for the development of this disorder?

3. What vital respiratory structure is destroyed by this condition?

4. How is this disease treated?

5. What is the role of a pulmonologist?

CHAPTER QUIZ

1. Along with the respiratory system, which system has the responsibility of supplying oxygen and eliminating carbon dioxide?

   a. muscular
   b. cardiovascular
   c. nervous
   d. integumentary
   e. none of the above

Answer:

2. The lacrimal ducts empty into the

   a. nose
   b. mouth
   c. throat
   d. trachea
   e. none of the above

Answer:

3. The nasal septum is made of

   a. epithelial tissue
   b. tendons
   c. bone

   d. cartilage
   e. none of the above

Answer:

4. Which of the following is NOT a function of the vestibules?

   a. warm incoming air
   b. smell
   c. filter air

   d. help create speech sounds
   e. peristalsis

Answer:

5. Olfactory receptors are located in the

   a. superior meatus
   b. middle meatus
   c. inferior meatus

   d. oropharynx
   e. none of the above

Answer:

6. Microorganisms that enter with air and are filtered out are destroyed by

   a. cilia
   b. mucus
   c. enzymes and acid

   d. hairs
   e. none of the above

Answer:

7. The pharynx is divided into how many portions?

   a. 2
   b. 3
   c. 4

   d. 5
   e. none of the above

Answer:

8. Which portion of the pharynx connects with the esophagus?

   a. eustachian tube
   b. oropharynx
   c. nasopharynx

   d. laryngopharynx
   e. none of the above

Answer:

9. Which of the following is a single cartilage in the larynx?

   a. thyroid
   b. cuneiform
   c. arytenoid

   d. corniculate
   e. none of the above

Answer:

10. Which of the following cartilages is rod shaped?

    a. cricoid
    b. arytenoid
    c. corniculate

    d. thyroid
    e. none of the above

Answer:

11. Together with the epiglottis, which of the following helps to keep food or liquids from entering the larynx?

    a. corniculate cartilage

    b. cuneiform cartilage

    c. vestibular folds

    d. vocal folds

    e. none of the above

Answer:

12. Which of the following structures function as resonating chambers?

    a. pharynx

    b. mouth

    c. nasal cavities

    d. paranasal sinuses

    e. all of the above

Answer:

13. Where does the trachea divide into left and right primary bronchi?

    a. cricoid cartilage

    b. fifth thoracic vertebra

    c. arytenoid cartilage

    d. fifth cervical vertebra

    e. none of the above

Answer:

14. If the C-shaped incomplete rings of cartilage in the trachea were complete closed rings, what would you NOT be able to do?

    a. inhale

    b. eat

    c. swallow

    d. talk

    e. exhale

Answer:

15. If a foreign object gets by the trachea, it would most likely get caught in the

    a. right primary bronchus

    b. left primary bronchus

    c. secondary bronchi

    d. tertiary bronchi

    e. none of the above

Answer:

16. Which of the bronchi are segmented?

    a. right primary

    b. left primary

    c. secondary

    d. tertiary

    e. none of the above

Answer:

17. The lungs are

    a. rod shaped

    b. wedge shaped

    c. leaf shaped

    d. cone shaped

    e. none of the above

Answer:

18. The right lung has how many lobes?

    a. 1
    b. 2
    c. 3

    d. 4
    e. none of the above

Answer:

19. The left lung has how many lobes?

    a. 1
    b. 2
    c. 3

    d. 4
    e. none of the above

Answer:

20. Which does a lobule NOT contain?

    a. lymphatic vessel
    b. a venule
    c. an arteriole

    d. bronchioles
    e. pleura

Answer:

21. Atria are found in the

    a. bronchopulmonary segment
    b. alveolar ducts
    c. alveoli

    d. segmented bronchi
    e. none of the above

Answer:

22. The third process of respiration is

    a. inhalation
    b. external respiration
    c. internal respiration

    d. exhalation
    e. none of the above

Answer:

23. Destruction of the walls of the alveoli occurs in which disease?

    a. emphysema
    b. bronchitis
    c. cystic fibrosis

    d. pulmonary fibrosis
    e. none of the above

Answer:

24. The disease common in infants is

    a. emphysema
    b. pulmonary fibrosis
    c. hyaline membrane disease

    d. pertussis
    e. none of the above

Answer:

25. Which of the following is an inherited disease?

    a. cystic fibrosis
    b. pulmonary fibrosis
    c. hyaline membrane disease

    d. pertussis
    e. none of the above

Answer:

26. Which of the following is a chronic bacterial infection?

    a. influenza
    b. tuberculosis
    c. hyaline membrane disease

    d. SIDS
    e. none of the above

Answer:

27. Which of the following is caused by exposure to a gram-negative bacterium that produces an acute pneumonia?

    a. atelectasis
    b. lung cancer
    c. Legionnaires disease

    d. SIDS
    e. influenza

Answer:

28. Which of the following is the most common cause of cancer deaths in the United States?

    a. lung cancer
    b. mouth cancer
    c. throat cancer

    d. nasal cancer
    e. gastric cancer

Answer:

The Urinary System

OBJECTIVES

After studying this chapter, you should be able to:

1. Define the function of the urinary system.

2. Name the external layers of the kidney.

3. Define the following internal parts of the kidneys: cortex, medulla, medullary pyramids, renal papillae, renal columns, and major and minor calyces.

4. Name the parts of a nephron, and describe the flow of urine throughout this renal tubule.

5. List the functions of the nephrons.

6. Explain how urine flows down the ureters.

7. Describe micturition and the role of stretch receptors in the bladder.

8. Compare the length and course of the male urethra to the female urethra.

9. Name the normal constituents of urine.

ACTIVITIES

A. Completion

Fill in the blank spaces with the correct term.

1. The urinary system consists of two ___, two ___, one ___, and one ___.

2. The kidneys are crucial in maintaining ___.

3. If kidney failure occurs, medical treatment consists of ___.

NAME: _____   DATE: _____

4. The elimination of wastes by the kidneys is called ___.

5. The kidneys regulate the concentration of ___ in body fluids and blood.

6. The regulation of hydrogen ions is ___ regulation.

7. The enzyme renin helps regulate ___ ___.

8. The liver, the skin, and the kidneys all participate in the synthesis of ___.

9. The ureter leaves the kidney through the ___.

10. There are ___ layers of tissue surrounding each kidney.

11. The smooth, transparent, fibrous connective tissue membrane connecting with the outermost covering of the ureter is the ___ ___.

12. The mass of fatty tissue is the ___ ___.

13. The tips of the cortex are the ___ ___.

14. The cortex and the renal columns make up the ___ of the kidney.

15. The minor calyces collect ___.

16. Urine leaves the kidney through the ___.

17. The nephrons are the ___ units of the kidney.

18. The innermost layer of Bowman's glomerular capsule is made up of cells called ___.

19. The endothelial-capsular membrane is the site of ___ ___ and ___ ___ from the blood.

20. The part of Henle that is highly permeable to water and solutes is the ___ ___.

21. The kidney is supplied with blood from the left and right ___ ___.

22. About ___ of blood passes through the kidneys every minute.

23. The interlobar arteries are found in the ___ ___.

24. The nerve supply to the kidney comes from the ___ ___.

25. The process that transports substances out of the tubular fluid and back into the blood is ___ ___.

26. The bladder wall has three layers of smooth muscle known as the ___ muscle.

27. Micturition is precipitated by ___ ___.

28. Urine in the urethra is transported by ___.

29. ___ is caused by a high concentration of uric acid in the plasma.

30. ___ is an inflammation of the urinary bladder.

31. ___ ___ can result from almost any condition that interferes with kidney function.

32. Urinary ___ is a condition in which an individual experiences an uncontrollable and continued flow of urine.

33. The kidneys produce ___, a hormone that stimulates red blood cell production.

B. Matching

Match the term on the right with the definition on the left.

_____ 34. helps adjust filtration pressure   a. parenchyma

_____ 35. kidney cavity   b. Bowman's capsule

_____ 36. inner layer around the kidney   c. glomerulus

_____ 37. outer layer around the kidney

_____ 38. striated triangular structure

_____ 39. point toward the kidney center

_____ 40. cortex and renal pyramids

_____ 41. collecting funnel

_____ 42. double-walled globe

_____ 43. Bowman's capsule and glomerulus

_____ 44. U-shaped structure

_____ 45. capillary network in the kidney

_____ 46. smooth muscle in the bladder wall

_____ 47. caused by uric acid in plasma

_____ 48. helps regulate urine production

d. renal corpuscle

e. loop of Henle

f. detrusor muscle

g. gout

h. aldosterone

i. renal pyramids

j. renal papillae

k. renal sinus

l. renin

m. renal pelvis

n. renal capsule

o. renal fascia

C. Key Terms

Use the text to look up the following terms. Write the definition or explanation.

49. Adipose capsule:

_____

_____

50. Afferent arteriole:

_____

_____

51. Arcuate arteries:

_____

_____

52. Arcuate veins:

_____

_____

53. Ascending limb of Henle:

_____

_____

54. Bowman's glomerular capsule:

_____

_____

55. Collecting duct:

_____

_____

56. Cortex:

_____

_____

57. Descending limb of Henle:

_____

_____

58. Detrusor muscle:

_____

_____

59. Distal convoluted tubule:

_____

_____

60. Efferent arteriole:

_____

_____

61. Endothelial-capsular membrane:

_____

_____

62. Erythropoietin:

_____

_____

63. External urinary sphincter:

_____

_____

64. Glomerulus:

_____

_____

65. Hilum:

_____

_____

66. Interlobular arteries:

_____

_____

67. Interlobular veins:

_____

_____

68. Internal urinary sphincter:

_____

_____

69. Kidney:

_____

_____

70. Kidney stones:

_____

_____

71. Left renal artery:

_____

_____

72. Left renal vein:

_____

_____

73. Loop of Henle:

_____

_____

74. Major calyces:

_____

_____

75. Medulla:

_____

_____

76. Micturition:

_____

_____

77. Micturition reflex:

_____

_____

78. Minor calyx:

_____

_____

79. Nephrons:

_____

_____

80. Oliguria:

_____

_____

81. Papillary ducts:

_____

_____

82. Parenchyma:

_____

_____

83. Peritubular capillaries:

_____

_____

84. Podocytes:

_____

_____

85. Proximal convoluted tubule:

_____

_____

86. Renal capsule:

_____

_____

87. Renal columns:

_____

_____

88. Renal corpuscle:

_____

_____

89. Renal fascia:

_____

_____

90. Renal papillae:

_____

_____

91. Renal pelvis:

_____

_____

92. Renal plexus:

_____

_____

93. Renal pyramids:

_____

_____

94. Renal sinus:

_____

_____

95. Renal tubule:

_____

_____

96. Renin:

_____

_____

97. Right renal artery:

_____

_____

98. Right renal vein:

_____

_____

99. Trigone:

_____

_____

100. Ureter:

_____

_____

101. Urethra:

_____

_____

102. Urinary bladder:

_____

_____

103. Urinary system:

_____

_____

104. Urine:

_____

_____

D. Labeling Exercise

105. Label the parts of the urinary system as indicated in Figure 18-1.

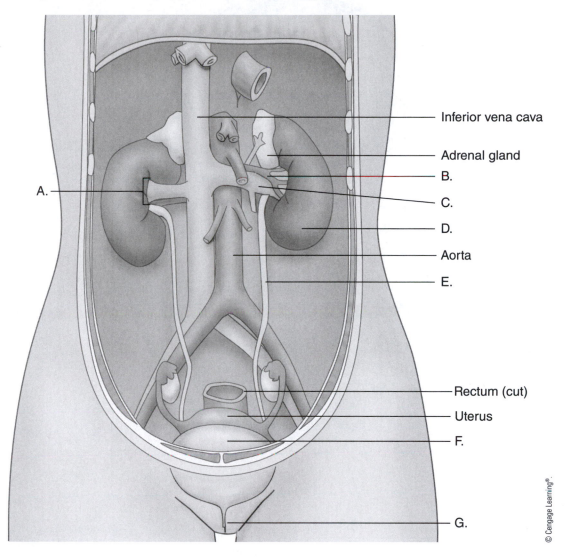

Inferior vena cava

Adrenal gland

B.

C.

D.

Aorta

E.

Rectum (cut)

Uterus

F.

G.

A.

© Cengage Learning®.

Figure 18-1

A. _____

B. _____

C. _____

D. _____

E. _____

F. _____

G. _____

106. Label the parts of the kidney as indicated in Figure 18-2.

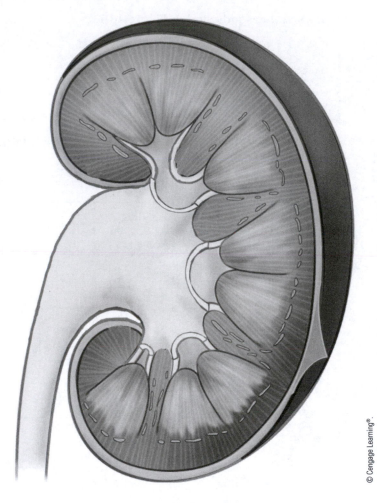

Figure 18-2

A. _____

B. _____

C. _____

D. _____

E. _____

F. _____

G. _____

H. _____

E. Coloring Exercise

107. Using Figure 18-3, color the proximal convoluted tubule, the distal convoluted tubule, and the loop of Henle orange; the interlobar artery and the afferent arteriole red; the interlobar vein blue; and the collecting duct yellow.

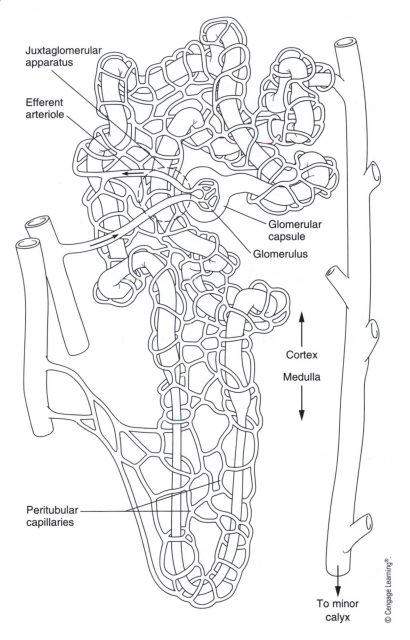

Juxtaglomerular apparatus

Efferent arteriole

Glomerular capsule

Glomerulus

Cortex

Medulla

Peritubular capillaries

To minor calyx

© Cengage Learning®.

Figure 18-2

F. Critical Thinking

Answer the following questions in complete sentences.

108. How do the kidneys help to maintain homeostasis?

109. How do the kidneys compensate for excessive perspiration?

110. Explain the part the kidneys play in the regulation of erythrocyte concentration.

111. Describe the role of the kidneys in teeth and bone development.

112. Why isn't hemodialysis a perfect substitute for kidney function?

113. Explain renal calculi and their treatment.

114. How does the endocrine system aid the kidneys to maintain homeostasis?

115. Explain why it can be said that the effects of aging on the urinary system begin as early as age 20.

116. Differentiate between a urologist and a nephrologist.

G. Crossword Puzzle

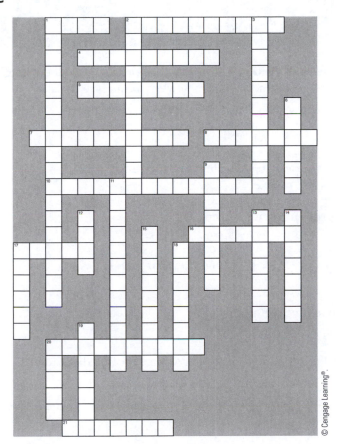

Complete the crossword puzzle using the following clues.

ACROSS

1. High uric acid in plasma

2. Cortex and renal pyramids

4. Waste elimination

5. Urinary bladder inflammation

DOWN

1. Kidney inflammation

2. Capillaries form interlobar vein

3. Voiding

6. Outer kidney area

7. Capillary network surrounded by podocytes

8. Transports urine by peristalsis

10. Stimulates red blood cell production

16. Veins connecting to interlobar veins

17. Formed by three processes in nephrons

20. Active vitamin D

21. Smooth triangular region of bladder

9. Functional units of kidneys

11. Procedure that filters blood

12. Transformed from ammonia by liver

13. Kidney stones

14. Inner kidney area

15. Visceral layer of Bowman's capsule

17. Transports urine to the bladder

18. Three layers of bladder wall smooth muscle

19. Stores urine

20. Collects urine from renal pyramids

C A S E   S T U D Y

Colleen, a 28-year-old woman, is visiting her health care provider. Colleen states she has pain and burning when she urinates as well as the need to urinate very frequently. This morning she saw what appeared to be blood in her urine.

QUESTIONS

1. Why might Colleen be experiencing burning and pain upon urination as well as frequency?

2. What might be causing the problem?

3. Why are women at greater risk for this condition than men?

4. How is this condition usually treated?

5. What measures can both men and women take to prevent this disorder?

CHAPTER QUIZ

1. A scant amount of urine is called

   a. hematuria
   b. polyuria
   c. oliguria

   d. pyuria
   e. none of the above

Answer:

2. Pus in the urine is called

    a. hematuria
    b. polyuria
    c. oliguria

    d. pyuria
    e. none of the above

Answer:

3. Urine in the blood is called

    a. hematuria
    b. polyuria
    c. oliguria

    d. pyuria
    e. none of the above

Answer:

4. Hemodialysis is the same as

    a. hematuria
    b. polyuria
    c. oliguria

    d. pyuria
    e. none of the above

Answer:

5. Besides the urinary system, which system controls urine production and micturition?

    a. muscular
    b. endocrine
    c. nervous

    d. integumentary
    e. none of the above

Answer:

6. Which system besides the urinary system is involved in the production of vitamin D?

    a. muscular
    b. endocrine
    c. nervous

    d. integumentary
    e. none of the above

Answer:

7. Urea is the product of the liver breaking down

    a. water
    b. ammonia
    c. sugar

    d. starch
    e. none of the above

Answer:

8. Urine formation begins with the process of

    a. micturition
    b. glomerular filtration
    c. tubular reabsorption

    d. tubular secretion
    e. none of the above

Answer:

9. How much of the kidney can be nonfunctional and still keep the person alive?

    a. ⅔
    b. ½
    c. ⅓

    d. ¾
    e. none of the above

Answer:

10. The regulation of pH is the control of which ions?

    a. hydrogen
    b. potassium
    c. calcium

    d. sodium
    e. none of the above

Answer:

11. The active form of vitamin D is

    a. calcium
    b. calciferol
    c. chloride

    d. sodium
    e. none of the above

Answer:

12. The innermost layer of the kidney is the

    a. renal sinus
    b. hilum
    c. renal capsule

    d. renal fascia
    e. none of the above

Answer:

13. The part of the kidney consisting of connective tissue and fat is the

    a. renal sinus
    b. hilum
    c. renal capsule

    d. renal fascia
    e. none of the above

Answer:

14. The part of the kidney that anchors it is the

    a. renal sinus
    b. hilum
    c. renal capsule

    d. renal fascia
    e. none of the above

Answer:

15. The millions of microscopic collecting tubules make up the

    a. nephron
    b. parenchyma
    c. pyramids

    d. cortex
    e. none of the above

Answer:

16. In the ducts of the pyramids, urine is directly collected by the

    a. nephrons
    b. minor calyces
    c. major calyces

    d. ureter
    e. none of the above

Answer:

17. Podocytes make up which layer of Bowman's glomerular capsule?

    a. visceral
    b. parietal
    c. outer

    d. cortex
    e. none of the above

Answer:

18. The visceral layer of Bowman's capsule and the endothelial capillary network make up a(n)

    a. vein
    b. capsule
    c. endothelial-capsular membrane
    d. tubule
    e. none of the above

Answer:

19. The papillary ducts empty into the

    a. renal capsule
    b. renal pelvis
    c. renal fascia
    d. pyramids
    e. none of the above

Answer:

20. Those materials in the blood responsible for the acid or alkaline components of the blood are

    a. salts
    b. sugars
    c. electrolytes
    d. plasma
    e. none of the above

Answer:

21. The renal artery divides into several branches that enter the parenchyma. In the renal columns, they are called

    a. interlobar arteries
    b. arcuate arteries
    c. interlobular arteries
    d. efferent arteries
    e. none of the above

Answer:

22. Glomerular capillaries unite and form the

    a. interlobar arteries
    b. arcuate arteries
    c. interlobular arteries
    d. efferent arteries
    e. none of the above

Answer:

23. The peritubular capillaries form the

    a. arcuate vein
    b. interlobular vein
    c. interlobar vein
    d. efferent vein
    e. none of the above

Answer:

24. The kidney's nerve supply comes from the

    a. central nervous system
    b. peripheral nervous system
    c. parasympathetic system
    d. sympathetic system
    e. none of the above

Answer:

25. The process responsible for regulating pH in the blood is called

    a. tubular secretion
    b. glomerular filtration
    c. micturition
    d. tubular reabsorption
    e. none of the above

Answer:

26. Increased blood pressure is a result of

    a. tubular formation
    b. glomerular filtration
    c. tubular reabsorption

    d. tubular secretion
    e. none of the above

Answer:

27. The daily production of urine depends on

    a. fluid intake
    b. temperature
    c. humidity

    d. emotional state
    e. all of the above

Answer:

28. The detrusor muscle consists of how many layers?

    a. 1
    b. 2
    c. 3

    d. 4
    e. none of the above

Answer:

29. The stretch receptors in the bladder begin to send messages when there is how much urine in the bladder?

    a. 700–800 mL
    b. 500–600 mL
    c. 400–600 mL

    d. 200–400 mL
    e. none of the above

Answer:

30. Which of the following can become acute following strep throat?

    a. cystitis
    b. gout
    c. glomerulonephritis

    d. glycosuria
    e. none of the above

Answer:

31. By age 80, what proportion of the kidney's glomeruli has ceased to function?

    a. ¼
    b. ⅓
    c. ½

    d. ⅔
    e. ⅘

Answer:

32. Which form of polycystic kidney disease is characterized by lower back pain and high blood pressure?

    a. adult
    b. childhood
    c. congenital

    d. pancreatic
    e. renal

Answer:

33. Which of the following species of bacterium commonly causes UTIs?

    a. *S. aureus*
    b. *M. tuberculosis*
    c. *S. pneumoniae*

    d. *E. coli*
    e. none of the above

Answer:

CHAPTER 19

The Reproductive System

OBJECTIVES

After studying this chapter, you should be able to:

1. Name the internal parts of a testis.
2. Explain the effects of testosterone on the male body.
3. Describe the process of spermatogenesis.
4. Follow the path of a sperm from the seminiferous tubules to the outside.
5. Define *semen* and what glands contribute to its composition.
6. Name the three parts of the male urethra.
7. Describe the development of a follicle before and after ovulation.
8. Describe the process of oogenesis.
9. Name the parts of the uterus.
10. Name the external genitalia of the female.
11. Describe the phases of the menstrual cycle.
12. Describe lactation and the function of the mammary glands.
13. Name the phases of labor.

ACTIVITIES

A. Completion

Fill in the blank spaces with the correct term.

1. Cell division resulting in 23 chromosomes in the egg and sperm is called ___.

NAME: _____   DATE: _____

2. Immediately following the union of sperm and egg, the fertilized egg is designated a(n) ___.

3. When producing sperm, the testes are considered ___ glands.

4. When the testes are producing the hormone testosterone, they are ___ glands.

5. The testes are raised and lowered in reaction to changes in ___.

6. The inside of the scrotum has ___ sacs; these sacs are separated by a(n) ___.

7. The ___ ___ extends inward and divides the testes into small compartments called lobules.

8. In the testicular lobules are found the ___ ___.

9. Meiosis occurs in the ___ ___.

10. Sertoli cells provide ___ for the sperm, and the interstitial cells of Leydig produce ___.

11. The acrosome contains ___, which help the sperm penetrate the ovum.

12. Mitochondria provide energy for the ___ of the sperm, which propels it on its journey.

13. The straight tubules lead to the ___ ___.

14. The sperm leave the testes through the efferent ducts and enter the ___ ___.

15. The seminal duct is another name for the ___ ___.

16. The part of the urethra found in the penis is the ___ urethra.

17. Three sets of accessory glands add secretions to the semen. The ones contributing the most are the ___ ___.

18. Protection of the sperm against bacteria is the function of ___.

19. As exocrine glands, the ovaries produce ___, and as endocrine glands they produce ___ and ___.

20. The ___ of the ovary contains ovarian follicles.

21. An egg is an ovum and an immature egg is a(n) ___.

22. After the egg is ejected from the follicle, the follicle becomes the ___ ___.

23. The total number of eggs a woman can produce is determined at ___.

24. It is in the primary oocytes that ___ occurs.

25. It is the very small cell called the ___ ___ that is nonfunctional.

26. The funnel-shaped opening at the end of each fallopian tube is called the ___.

27. Fertilization takes place in the ___ ___.

28. The ___ ___ is the opening of the cervix into the vagina.

29. The visceral peritoneum of the uterus is a serous membrane known as the ___.

30. During the menstrual phase, a clear membrane called the ___ ___ develops around the eggs.

31. The ovum is not released directly into the uterine tube but into the ___ ___.

32. The beginning and end of the menstrual cycle in a woman's life are called ___ and ___.

33. The recess surrounding the vaginal attachment to the cervix is called the ___.

34. The mons pubis is also called the ___.

35. The ___ ___ of the external genitalia contain numerous sebaceous glands.

36. The glands homologous to the male Cowper's glands are the ___ glands.

37. The size of the breast is determined by the amount of ___ ___.

38. Human chorionic gonadotropin (hCG) is secreted by the ___ ___.

39. At the ninth week, the embryo is known as a(n) ___.

40. ___ is the name given to childbirth.

41. The scrotum is an outpouching of the ___ ___.

42. The most common ectopic pregnancies occur in the ___ ___.

43. Male infertility is most commonly caused by a low ___ ___ count.

B. Matching

Match the term on the right with the definition on the left.

____ 44. cellular division that produces sex cells   a. fallopian tubes

____ 45. elevates the testes   b. Sertoli cells

____ 46. connective tissue covering the testes   c. myometrium

____ 47. daughter cells   d. graafian follicle

____ 48. supply nutrients for sperm   e. foreskin

____ 49. produced by the interstitial cells of Leydig   f. cremaster muscle

____ 50. where sperm cells mature   g. germinal epithelium

____ 51. secrete alkaline mucus   h. corpus luteum

____ 52. penis head   i. corpus albicans

____ 53. prepuce   j. Cowper's glands

____ 54. covers the surface of the ovary   k. primary spermatocytes

____ 55. mature follicle with the mature egg   l. vulva

____ 56. white body   m. epididymis

____ 57. transport eggs to the uterus   n. mons pubis

____ 58. between the body and cervix   o. tunica albuginea

____ 59. uterine middle layer   p. meiosis

____ 60. yellow body   q. lactation

____ 61. external female genitalia   r. glans penis

____ 62. veneris   s. testosterone

____ 63. secrete and eject milk   t. isthmus

C. Key Terms

Use the text to look up the following words. Write the definition or explanation.

64. Acrosome:

_____

_____

65. Alveoli:

_____

_____

66. Amnion:

_____

_____

67. Ampullae/lactiferous sinuses:

_____

_____

68. Areola:

_____

_____

69. Blastula/blastocyst:

_____

_____

70. Body of the uterus:

_____

_____

71. Bulbourethral/Cowper's glands:

_____

_____

72. Cervical canal:

_____

_____

73. Cervix:

_____

_____

74. Chorionic vesicle:

_____

_____

75. Chorionic villi:

_____

_____

76. Clitoris:

_____

_____

77. Coitus:

_____

_____

78. Corpus albicans:

_____

_____

79. Corpus hemorrhagicum:

_____

_____

80. Corpus luteum:

_____

_____

81. Cremaster muscle:

_____

_____

82. Ductus (vas) deferens:

_____

_____

83. Ductus epididymis:

_____

_____

84. Ectoderm:

_____

_____

85. Efferent ducts:

_____

_____

86. Ejaculatory duct:

_____

_____

87. Endoderm:

_____

_____

88. Endometrium:

_____

_____

89. Erection:

_____

_____

90. Estrogen:

_____

_____

91. External os:

_____

_____

92. Fetus:

_____

_____

93. Fimbriae:

_____

_____

94. Fornix:

_____

_____

95. Fundus:

_____

_____

96. Germinal epithelium:

_____

_____

97. Glans:

_____

_____

98. Glans penis:

_____

_____

99. Graafian follicle:

_____

_____

100. Greater vestibular/Bartholin's glands:

_____

_____

101. Hymen:

_____

_____

102. Infundibulum:

_____

_____

103. Internal os:

_____

_____

104. Interstitial cells of Leydig:

_____

_____

105. Isthmus:

_____

_____

106. Labia majora:

_____

_____

107. Labia minora:

_____

_____

108. Labor:

_____

_____

109. Lactation:

_____

_____

110. Lactiferous ducts:

_____

_____

111. Lesser vestibular/Skene's glands:

_____

_____

112. Mammary glands:

_____

_____

113. Membranous urethra:

_____

_____

114. Menarche:

_____

_____

115. Menopause:

_____

_____

116. Menses:

_____

_____

117. Menstrual cycle:

_____

_____

118. Menstruation:

_____

_____

119. Mesoderm:

_____

_____

120. Mons pubis/veneris:

_____

_____

121. Myometrium:

_____

_____

122. Nipple:

_____

_____

123. Oocyte:

_____

_____

124. Oogenesis:

_____

_____

125. Oogonia:

_____

_____

126. Ootid:

_____

_____

127. Ova:

_____

_____

128. Ovarian cycle:

_____

_____

129. Ovarian follicles:

_____

_____

130. Ovaries:

_____

_____

131. Ovulation:

_____

_____

132. Parturition:

_____

_____

133. Penis:

_____

_____

134. Perimetrium:

_____

_____

135. Perineum:

_____

_____

136. Phimosis:

_____

_____

137. Placenta:

_____

_____

138. Polar body:

_____

_____

139. Prepuce/foreskin:

_____

_____

140. Primary oocytes:

_____

_____

141. Primary spermatocytes:

_____

_____

142. Progesterone:

_____

_____

143. Prostate gland:

_____

_____

144. Prostatic urethra:

_____

_____

145. Raphe:

_____

_____

146. Rete testis:

_____

_____

147. Scrotum:

_____

_____

148. Secondary oocyte:

_____

_____

149. Secondary spermatocytes:

_____

_____

150. Semen/seminal fluid:

_____

_____

151. Seminal vesicles:

_____

_____

152. Seminalplasmin:

_____

_____

153. Seminiferous tubules:

_____

_____

154. Sertoli cells:

_____

_____

155. Shaft:

_____

_____

156. Spermatic cord:

_____

_____

157. Spermatids:

_____

_____

158. Spermatogenesis:

_____

_____

159. Spermatogonia:

_____

_____

160. Spermatozoa:

_____

_____

161. Spongy/cavernous urethra:

_____

_____

162. Straight tubules:

_____

_____

163. Testes:

_____

_____

164. Testosterone:

_____

_____

165. Tunica albuginea:

_____

_____

166. Umbilical cord:

_____

_____

167. Urethra:

_____

_____

168. Urethral orifice:

_____

_____

169. Uterine cavity:

_____

_____

170. Uterine/fallopian tubes:

_____

_____

171. Uterus:

_____

_____

172. Vagina:

_____

_____

173. Vaginal orifice:

_____

_____

174. Vasectomy:

_____

_____

175. Vestibule:

_____

_____

176. Vulva/pudendum:

_____

_____

177. Zygote:

_____

_____

D. Labeling Exercise

178. Label the parts of the male reproductive system as indicated in Figure 19-1.

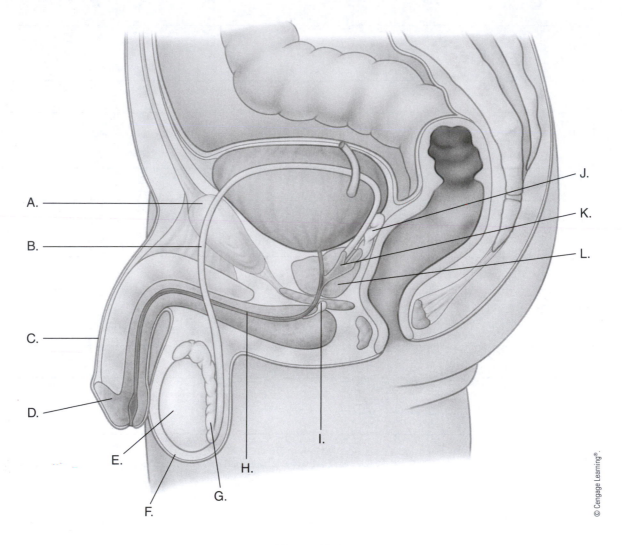

Figure 19-1

A. _____   G. _____

B. _____   H. _____

C. _____   I. _____

D. _____   J. _____

E. _____   K. _____

F. _____   L. _____

179. Label the parts of the female reproductive system as indicated in Figure 19-2.

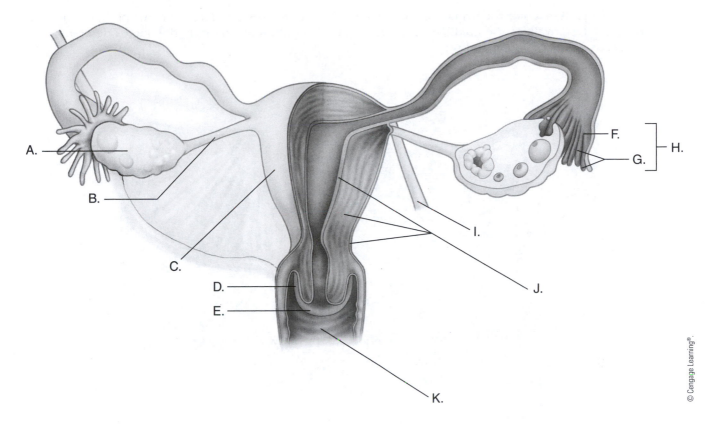

Figure 19-2

A. _____   G. _____

B. _____   H. _____

C. _____   I. _____

D. _____   J. _____

E. _____   K. _____

F. _____

E. Coloring Exercise

180. Using Figure 19-3, color the urinary bladder green, the seminal vesicle blue, the penis pink, the urethra green, the testis yellow, the epididymis brown, the bulbourethral gland black, the ductus deferens orange, and the prostate gland red.

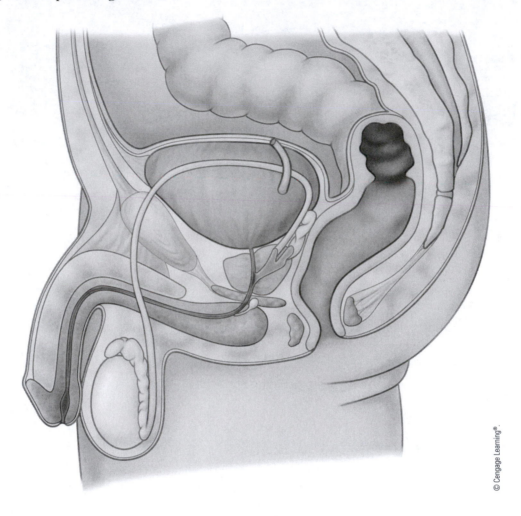

Figure 19-3

181. Using Figure 19-4, color the pectoralis major muscle red, the adipose tissue yellow, the lactiferous sinus green, the nipple pink, and the areola brown.

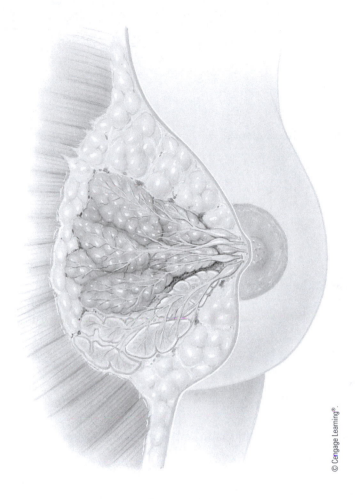

Figure 19-4

F. Critical Thinking

Answer the following questions in complete sentences.

182. Why are meiosis and mitosis so important to human reproduction?

183. Explain why it is so important for a pregnant woman to refrain from taking drugs and alcohol and maintain a proper diet.

184. Explain the significance of the placenta.

185. What is the difference in the supply of the ova and sperm?

186. Explain the difference between sterility and impotence.

187. Describe the functions of the male accessory reproductive glands.

188. As women age, a primary change is the onset of menopause. What changes happen to men?

189. Distinguish between a gynecologist and an obstetrician.

190. Distinguish between a pediatrician and a neonatalist.

G. Crossword Puzzle

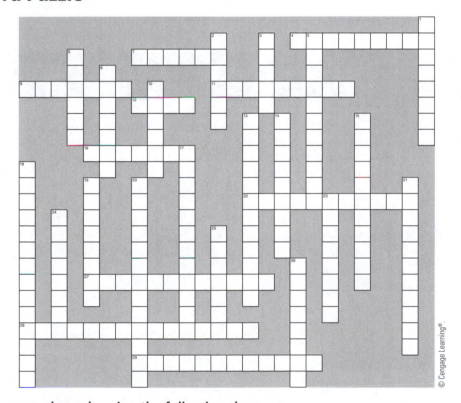

Complete the crossword puzzle using the following clues.

ACROSS

4. Last menstrual cycle
7. Fertilized egg
9. Sore caused by primary stage of syphilis
11. Male birth control procedure

DOWN

1. First menstrual cycle
2. Uterine opening to the vagina
3. Sperm and secretions
5. Uterine inner layer

12. Uterus

16. Supporting structure of the testes

22. Mature sperm cells

27. Male hormone

28. Produce sperm

29. Funnel-shaped open end to the fallopian tube

6. Fluid-filled sac surrounding the embryo

8. Foreskin of the penis

10. Immature egg

13. Female hormone

14. Egg formation occurring in the ovaries

15. Flagellate protozoan

17. Cyclical shedding of the lining of the uterus

18. Semen antibiotic

19. Secretes alkaline fluid

20. Immature sperm cells

21. Childbirth

23. Contains enzymes that aid sperm in penetration

24. Finger-like projections around the infundibulum

25. Female gonads

26. Vulva

CASE STUDY

Jahdai, a 27-year-old man, visits a public health clinic with complaints of burning on urination, and the occasional discharge of pus from his penis. He tells the health care provider that he had unprotected sex with a partner approximately 1 week ago. The health care provider assesses Jahdai's genital area and notes a small discharge of pus from the uretheral orifice.

QUESTIONS

1. What condition do you think might be causing Jahdai's symptoms?

2. What causes this condition?

3. How do the symptoms of this disorder manifest in men as opposed to women?

4. How will Jahdai's problem be treated?

5. What measures can people take to prevent this disorder?

CHAPTER QUIZ

1. A highly contagious infectious disease caused by a virus is

   a. genital warts
   b. syphilis
   c. genital herpes

   d. trichomonas
   e. gonorrhea

Answer:

2. Which is caused by a bacterium and has several stages?

   a. genital warts
   b. syphilis
   c. genital herpes

   d. trichomonas
   e. gonorrhea

Answer:

3. Which is caused by a flagellate protozoan and is more common in females?

   a. genital warts
   b. syphilis
   c. genital herpes

   d. trichomonas
   e. gonorrhea

Answer:

4. A viral infection causing lesions and blister-like eruptions is

   a. genital warts
   b. syphilis
   c. genital herpes

   d. trichomonas
   e. gonorrhea

Answer:

5. When the foreskin of the penis fits too tightly over the head, it is called

   a. pelvic inflammatory disease
   b. PMS
   c. gonorrhea

   d. phimosis
   e. trichomonas

Answer:

6. Which bacterial infection invades the epithelial lining of the vagina and male urethra?

   a. pelvic inflammatory disease
   b. PMS
   c. gonorrhea

   d. phimosis
   e. trichomonas

Answer:

7. A bacterial infection of the uterus, uterine tubes, and/or ovaries is

   a. pelvic inflammatory disease
   b. PMS
   c. gonorrhea

   d. phimosis
   e. trichomonas

Answer:

8. The process producing sperm is

    a. spermatogonia   d. spermatozoa
    b. spermatogenesis   e. none of the above
    c. spermatid

Answer:

9. The most immature sperm cells are

    a. spermatogonia   d. spermatozoa
    b. spermatogenesis   e. none of the above
    c. spermatid

Answer:

10. The most immature sperm cells divide by mitosis to produce daughter cells called

    a. spermatogonia   d. spermatozoa
    b. spermatogenesis   e. none of the above
    c. spermatid

Answer:

11. Secondary spermatocytes undergo a second meiotic division and become

    a. spermatogonia   d. spermatozoa
    b. spermatogenesis   e. none of the above
    c. spermatid

Answer:

12. Testosterone is produced by the

    a. Sertoli cells   d. spermatogonia cells
    b. sperm cells   e. none of the above
    c. interstitial cells of Leydig

Answer:

13. The enzyme aiding the sperm to penetrate the ovum is found in the

    a. tail   d. acrosome
    b. middle   e. none of the above
    c. skin

Answer:

14. Sperm cells are moved from the seminiferous tubules through the straight tubules to the

    a. rete testis   d. vas deferens
    b. efferent ducts   e. none of the above
    c. ductus epididymis

Answer:

15. The site of sperm storage while they mature is the

    a. rete testis   d. epididymis
    b. efferent ducts   e. none of the above
    c. straight tubules

Answer:

16. The portion of the urethra responsible for erection of the penis is the

    a. prostatic
    b. membranous
    c. cavernous

    d. bulb
    e. none of the above

Answer:

17. Which of the following is an accessory gland of the male reproductive system?

    a. ejaculatory duct
    b. seminal vesicles
    c. testis

    d. vas deferens
    e. none of the above

Answer:

18. Which of the following is also known as Cowper's?

    a. seminal vesicles
    b. ejaculatory duct
    c. prostate

    d. bulbourethral
    e. none of the above

Answer:

19. All of the following are accessory organs of the female reproductive system EXCEPT the

    a. fallopian tubes
    b. ovaries
    c. vagina

    d. Bartholin's gland
    e. vulva

Answer:

20. The ovaries are secured to the walls of the pelvis by

    a. ligaments
    b. tendons
    c. aponeurosis

    d. muscles
    e. none of the above

Answer:

21. The part of the ovary that produces estrogen and progesterone is known as the

    a. ovarian follicle
    b. secondary follicle
    c. corpus luteum

    d. graafian follicle
    e. none of the above

Answer:

22. During the second meiotic division, a mature egg cell is formed called a(n)

    a. oocyte
    b. ootid
    c. polar body

    d. oogonia
    e. none of the above

Answer:

23. If the female's egg is fertilized, where does it take place?

    a. the infundibulum
    b. the fimbriae
    c. uterine tube

    d. the uterus
    e. none of the above

Answer:

24. Which of the following is an anatomic division of the uterus?

    a. fundus
    b. body
    c. cervix

    d. isthmus
    e. all of the above

Answer:

25. The middle layer of the uterine wall is the

    a. myometrium
    b. endometrium
    c. ectometrium

    d. perimetrium
    e. none of the above

Answer:

26. The lining of the uterus that is shed during the menstrual cycle is the

    a. ectometrium
    b. endometrium
    c. myometrium

    d. perimetrium
    e. none of the above

Answer:

27. An egg or ovum is released during which phase of the menstrual cycle?

    a. menstrual
    b. proliferative or preovulatory
    c. postovulatory

    d. secretory
    e. none of the above

Answer:

28. Which is the following is a hormone related to pregnancy?

    a. luteinizing
    b. progesterone
    c. estrogen

    d. hCG
    e. all of the above

Answer:

29. All of the following are parts of the external genitalia EXCEPT

    a. mons pubis
    b. clitoris
    c. vestibular glands

    d. vagina
    e. vulva

Answer:

30. The portion of the female external genitalia that is homologous to the male penis is the

    a. labia minora
    b. mons pubis
    c. clitoris

    d. vestibule
    e. none of the above

Answer:

31. Which of the following can be caused by physically defective genitalia, type II diabetes, neuromuscular dysfunctions, or psychological issues?

    a. erectile dysfunction
    b. endometriosis
    c. ovarian cancer

    d. menstrual cramps
    e. none of the above

Answer:

32. Blockages of the fallopian tubes due to adhesions from various infections are the most common cause of

    a. endometriosis
    b. ovarian cancer
    c. impotence

    d. menstrual cramps
    e. female infertility

Answer:

33. Which phase of the menstrual cycle is the most constant in duration?

    a. menstrual
    b. preovulatory
    c. graafian

    d. postovulatory
    e. proliferative

Answer: